PASTEST POCKET SERIES FOR MRCP PART 1

BOOK 2
MCQs
IN
NEUROLOGY
AND
PSYCHIATRY

Edited by Richard L. Hawkins MBBS FRCS

Authors: C. M. C. Allen MA MD MRCP
Addenbrooke's Hospital,
Cambridge.

E. Gehlhaar BA MB MRCPsych
DGM
St Mary's Hospital, London.

D0988135

PASTEST

© 1987 PASTEST
Rankin House, Parkgate Estate,
Knutsford, Cheshire. WA16 8DX

First printed 1987
Reprinted 1988
Reprinted 1989
Reprinted 1991
Reprinted 1993

A catalogue record for this book is available from the
British Library.

ISBN: 0 906896 19 3

Text prepared by Turner Associates, Knutsford,
Cheshire.
Phototypeset by Communitype, Leicester
Printed by Martins The Printers, Berwick on Tweed

CONTENTS

INTRODUCTION

With more than twelve years of experience in postgraduate medical education to draw on, PASTEST have commissioned a series of reasonably priced MCQ books under the editorial mantle of Dr Richard Hawkins.

There is no better way to revise for the MRCP Part I examination than by answering good quality MCQs. These books, however, provide an additional dimension. The MCQs have been deliberately broken down by specialty and a self-assessment chart provided for each so that doctors can identify their strengths and weaknesses and plan their revision accordingly.

A significant number of questions in the MRCP Part I examination are devoted to Neurology and Psychiatry. This book provides approximately 50 representative questions from each specialty, with each question accompanied by a clear and simple explanatory answer. A strong emphasis on physiology, basic sciences and pharmacology has been included since the modern examination places such importance on these aspects.

The membership examination at present consists of sixty questions, each with a stem and five related questions: a total of 300 possible correct responses. Each correct response is awarded +1, each incorrect one -1, with no marks being awarded if the question is answered 'Don't know'. As in all examinations, proper technique can make the difference between a 'pass' and a 'bare fail'.

What, then, is the best approach? Firstly, the question stem must be read very carefully. Failure to notice a negative statement could result in a score of -5. In a 'close marked' examination this could quite easily be the difference between a pass and a fail. Secondly, the keywords used in MCQs should be identified: always/commonly/frequently/recognised/may/never, and so on. Each has a distinctly different meaning, thus: 'jaundice is a frequent complication of infectious mononucleosis' (false), whereas: 'jaundice may complicate infectious mononucleosis' (true). Beware of always and never.

Finally, answer those questions that you think you have a greater than 50% chance of getting correct. Thus, while leaving out questions in which you would be guessing (because in these you are likely to score 0 overall), do attempt those which you think you know something about; it is worth backing a hunch. Although your 'hit rate' will not be as high for these as for those questions for which you think you know the answer, overall you will score positively. Candidates do fail because they do not attempt enough questions, and it is worth remembering that even some of those answers that you are confident about may, in fact, be wrong.

Time for revision is often at a premium because preparation has to be done at the same time as a busy medical SHO job. A few general tips may be useful:

1. Do not read systematically through large medical textbooks, but rather base your revision around multiple choice questions. The self-assessment charts provided in this book may be helpful here. Direct further reading of standard texts to those areas in which you are scoring low marks, in other words use these MCQs to identify 'blind spots' in your knowledge.

2. Make cards for those questions which come up frequently (such as modes of inheritance) and learn these.

3. A good course is probably worth the investment and your employer may be able to assist with the funding for this, if one is not provided at your hospital.

4. Aim to start your revision in good time and be sure you have time to cover most topics.

Cut-out self-assessment charts are included in this book so that you can record your answers to each MCQ as you work steadily through the questions. In order to give yourself a realistic time limit, do not spend more than 2 1/2 minutes on any one question. Some people may prefer to indicate their answers directly on the question pages in the spaces provided and then to transfer these answers on to the self-assessment charts. You can then correct your own answers against the answers given in the book and can calculate your total score in each section. By indicating clearly each item that you answered incorrectly you can then read the explanation provided and refer to a standard textbook for further revision on that topic.

Encyclopaedic specialist reference books are perhaps best avoided during preparation, only to be used for verification of detail. However, in the fields of neurology and psychiatry the following titles may be helpful:

Adams : **Principles of Neurology** (3rd edition). McGraw Hill.
Harrison, M.J.G. **Neurological skills**. Butterworth.
Matthews, W.B. **Disease of the Nervous System**. Blackwell.
Patten, J. **Neurological Differential Diagnosis**. H.Stark.
Bird and Harrison. **Examination Notes in Psychiatry**. Wright.
Gelder, Gath and Mayou. **Oxford Textbook of Psychiatry**. Oxford.

NEUROLOGY SELF-ASSESSMENT CHART

Please use 2B PENCIL only. Rub out all errors thoroughly.
Mark lozenges like ⬬ NOT like this ⊄ ⊄ ⊗

T ⬭ = TRUE F ⬭ = FALSE DK ⬭ = DON'T KNOW

	A	B	C	D	E
1	T F DK	T F DK	T F DK	T F DK	T F DK
2	T F DK	T F DK	T F DK	T F DK	T F DK
3	T F DK	T F DK	T F DK	T F DK	T F DK
4	T F DK	T F DK	T F DK	T F DK	T F DK
5	T F DK	T F DK	T F DK	T F DK	T F DK
6	T F DK	T F DK	T F DK	T F DK	T F DK
7	T F DK	T F DK	T F DK	T F DK	T F DK
8	T F DK	T F DK	T F DK	T F DK	T F DK
9	T F DK	T F DK	T F DK	T F DK	T F DK
10	T F DK	T F DK	T F DK	T F DK	T F DK
11	T F DK	T F DK	T F DK	T F DK	T F DK
12	T F DK	T F DK	T F DK	T F DK	T F DK
13	T F DK	T F DK	T F DK	T F DK	T F DK
14	T F DK	T F DK	T F DK	T F DK	T F DK
15	T F DK	T F DK	T F DK	T F DK	T F DK

	A	B	C	D	E
16	T F DK	T F DK	T F DK	T F DK	T F DK
17	T F DK	T F DK	T F DK	T F DK	T F DK
18	T F DK	T F DK	T F DK	T F DK	T F DK
19	T F DK	T F DK	T F DK	T F DK	T F DK
20	T F DK	T F DK	T F DK	T F DK	T F DK
21	T F DK	T F DK	T F DK	T F DK	T F DK
22	T F DK	T F DK	T F DK	T F DK	T F DK
23	T F DK	T F DK	T F DK	T F DK	T F DK
24	T F DK	T F DK	T F DK	T F DK	T F DK
25	T F DK	T F DK	T F DK	T F DK	T F DK
26	T F DK	T F DK	T F DK	T F DK	T F DK
27	T F DK	T F DK	T F DK	T F DK	T F DK
28	T F DK	T F DK	T F DK	T F DK	T F DK
29	T F DK	T F DK	T F DK	T F DK	T F DK
30	T F DK	T F DK	T F DK	T F DK	T F DK

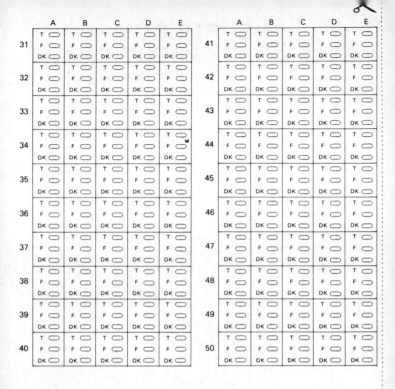

	A	B	C	D	E		A	B	C	D	E
31	T ⬭ F ⬭ DK ⬭	T ⬭ F ⬭ DK ⬭	T ⬭ F ⬭ DK ⬭	T ⬭ F ⬭ DK ⬭	T ⬭ F ⬭ DK ⬭	41	T ⬭ F ⬭ DK ⬭	T ⬭ F ⬭ DK ⬭	T ⬭ F ⬭ DK ⬭	T ⬭ F ⬭ DK ⬭	T ⬭ F ⬭ DK ⬭
32	T ⬭ F ⬭ DK ⬭	T ⬭ F ⬭ DK ⬭	T ⬭ F ⬭ DK ⬭	T ⬭ F ⬭ DK ⬭	T ⬭ F ⬭ DK ⬭	42	T ⬭ F ⬭ DK ⬭	T ⬭ F ⬭ DK ⬭	T ⬭ F ⬭ DK ⬭	T ⬭ F ⬭ DK ⬭	T ⬭ F ⬭ DK ⬭
33	T ⬭ F ⬭ DK ⬭	T ⬭ F ⬭ DK ⬭	T ⬭ F ⬭ DK ⬭	T ⬭ F ⬭ DK ⬭	T ⬭ F ⬭ DK ⬭	43	T ⬭ F ⬭ DK ⬭	T ⬭ F ⬭ DK ⬭	T ⬭ F ⬭ DK ⬭	T ⬭ F ⬭ DK ⬭	T ⬭ F ⬭ DK ⬭
34	T ⬭ F ⬭ DK ⬭	T ⬭ F ⬭ DK ⬭	T ⬭ F ⬭ DK ⬭	T ⬭ F ⬭ DK ⬭	T ⬭ F ⬭ DK ⬭	44	T ⬭ F ⬭ DK ⬭	T ⬭ F ⬭ DK ⬭	T ⬭ F ⬭ DK ⬭	T ⬭ F ⬭ DK ⬭	T ⬭ F ⬭ DK ⬭
35	T ⬭ F ⬭ DK ⬭	T ⬭ F ⬭ DK ⬭	T ⬭ F ⬭ DK ⬭	T ⬭ F ⬭ DK ⬭	T ⬭ F ⬭ DK ⬭	45	T ⬭ F ⬭ DK ⬭	T ⬭ F ⬭ DK ⬭	T ⬭ F ⬭ DK ⬭	T ⬭ F ⬭ DK ⬭	T ⬭ F ⬭ DK ⬭
36	T ⬭ F ⬭ DK ⬭	T ⬭ F ⬭ DK ⬭	T ⬭ F ⬭ DK ⬭	T ⬭ F ⬭ DK ⬭	T ⬭ F ⬭ DK ⬭	46	T ⬭ F ⬭ DK ⬭	T ⬭ F ⬭ DK ⬭	T ⬭ F ⬭ DK ⬭	T ⬭ F ⬭ DK ⬭	T ⬭ F ⬭ DK ⬭
37	T ⬭ F ⬭ DK ⬭	T ⬭ F ⬭ DK ⬭	T ⬭ F ⬭ DK ⬭	T ⬭ F ⬭ DK ⬭	T ⬭ F ⬭ DK ⬭	47	T ⬭ F ⬭ DK ⬭	T ⬭ F ⬭ DK ⬭	T ⬭ F ⬭ DK ⬭	T ⬭ F ⬭ DK ⬭	T ⬭ F ⬭ DK ⬭
38	T ⬭ F ⬭ DK ⬭	T ⬭ F ⬭ DK ⬭	T ⬭ F ⬭ DK ⬭	T ⬭ F ⬭ DK ⬭	T ⬭ F ⬭ DK ⬭	48	T ⬭ F ⬭ DK ⬭	T ⬭ F ⬭ DK ⬭	T ⬭ F ⬭ DK ⬭	T ⬭ F ⬭ DK ⬭	T ⬭ F ⬭ DK ⬭
39	T ⬭ F ⬭ DK ⬭	T ⬭ F ⬭ DK ⬭	T ⬭ F ⬭ DK ⬭	T ⬭ F ⬭ DK ⬭	T ⬭ F ⬭ DK ⬭	49	T ⬭ F ⬭ DK ⬭	T ⬭ F ⬭ DK ⬭	T ⬭ F ⬭ DK ⬭	T ⬭ F ⬭ DK ⬭	T ⬭ F ⬭ DK ⬭
40	T ⬭ F ⬭ DK ⬭	T ⬭ F ⬭ DK ⬭	T ⬭ F ⬭ DK ⬭	T ⬭ F ⬭ DK ⬭	T ⬭ F ⬭ DK ⬭	50	T ⬭ F ⬭ DK ⬭	T ⬭ F ⬭ DK ⬭	T ⬭ F ⬭ DK ⬭	T ⬭ F ⬭ DK ⬭	T ⬭ F ⬭ DK ⬭

CORRECT ANSWERS (+1) =

INCORRECT ANSWERS (−1) =

DON'T KNOW (0) _____

TOTAL SCORE: _____

(Maximum Score possible = 250)

PSYCHIATRY
SELF-ASSESSMENT CHART

Please use 2B PENCIL only. Rub out all errors thoroughly.
Mark lozenges like ▬ NOT like this ⊘ ⊘ ✗

T ⬭ = TRUE   F ⬭ = FALSE   DK ⬭ = DON'T KNOW

	A	B	C	D	E		A	B	C	D	E
51	T F DK	T F DK	T F DK	T F DK	T F DK	66	T F DK	T F DK	T F DK	T F DK	T F DK
52	T F DK	T F DK	T F DK	T F DK	T F DK	67	T F DK	T F DK	T F DK	T F DK	T F DK
53	T F DK	T F DK	T F DK	T F DK	T F DK	68	T F DK	T F DK	T F DK	T F DK	T F DK
54	T F DK	T F DK	T F DK	T F DK	T F DK	69	T F DK	T F DK	T F DK	T F DK	T F DK
55	T F DK	T F DK	T F DK	T F DK	T F DK	70	T F DK	T F DK	T F DK	T F DK	T F DK
56	T F DK	T F DK	T F DK	T F DK	T F DK	71	T F DK	T F DK	T F DK	T F DK	T F DK
57	T F DK	T F DK	T F DK	T F DK	T F DK	72	T F DK	T F DK	T F DK	T F DK	T F DK
58	T F DK	T F DK	T F DK	T F DK	T F DK	73	T F DK	T F DK	T F DK	T F DK	T F DK
59	T F DK	T F DK	T F DK	T F DK	T F DK	74	T F DK	T F DK	T F DK	T F DK	T F DK
60	T F DK	T F DK	T F DK	T F DK	T F DK	75	T F DK	T F DK	T F DK	T F DK	T F DK
61	T F DK	T F DK	T F DK	T F DK	T F DK	76	T F DK	T F DK	T F DK	T F DK	T F DK
62	T F DK	T F DK	T F DK	T F DK	T F DK	77	T F DK	T F DK	T F DK	T F DK	T F DK
63	T F DK	T F DK	T F DK	T F DK	T F DK	78	T F DK	T F DK	T F DK	T F DK	T F DK
64	T F DK	T F DK	T F DK	T F DK	T F DK	79	T F DK	T F DK	T F DK	T F DK	T F DK
65	T F DK	T F DK	T F DK	T F DK	T F DK	80	T F DK	T F DK	T F DK	T F DK	T F DK

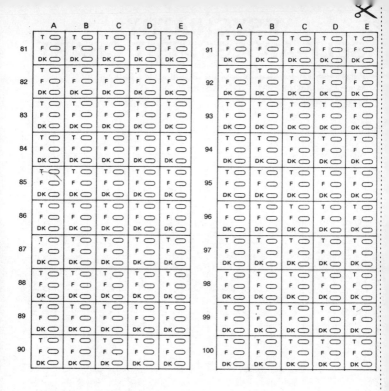

	A	B	C	D	E		A	B	C	D	E
81	T / F / DK	T / F / DK	T / F / DK	T / F / DK	T / F / DK	91	T / F / DK	T / F / DK	T / F / DK	T / F / DK	T / F / DK
82	T / F / DK	T / F / DK	T / F / DK	T / F / DK	T / F / DK	92	T / F / DK	T / F / DK	T / F / DK	T / F / DK	T / F / DK
83	T / F / DK	T / F / DK	T / F / DK	T / F / DK	T / F / DK	93	T / F / DK	T / F / DK	T / F / DK	T / F / DK	T / F / DK
84	T / F / DK	T / F / DK	T / F / DK	T / F / DK	T / F / DK	94	T / F / DK	T / F / DK	T / F / DK	T / F / DK	T / F / DK
85	T / F / DK	T / F / DK	T / F / DK	T / F / DK	T / F / DK	95	T / F / DK	T / F / DK	T / F / DK	T / F / DK	T / F / DK
86	T / F / DK	T / F / DK	T / F / DK	T / F / DK	T / F / DK	96	T / F / DK	T / F / DK	T / F / DK	T / F / DK	T / F / DK
87	T / F / DK	T / F / DK	T / F / DK	T / F / DK	T / F / DK	97	T / F / DK	T / F / DK	T / F / DK	T / F / DK	T / F / DK
88	T / F / DK	T / F / DK	T / F / DK	T / F / DK	T / F / DK	98	T / F / DK	T / F / DK	T / F / DK	T / F / DK	T / F / DK
89	T / F / DK	T / F / DK	T / F / DK	T / F / DK	T / F / DK	99	T / F / DK	T / F / DK	T / F / DK	T / F / DK	T / F / DK
90	T / F / DK	T / F / DK	T / F / DK	T / F / DK	T / F / DK	100	T / F / DK	T / F / DK	T / F / DK	T / F / DK	T / F / DK

CORRECT ANSWERS (+1)   =

INCORRECT ANSWERS (−1)   =

DON'T KNOW (0)   _____

TOTAL SCORE: _____

(Maximum Score possible = 250)

X

Indicate your answers by putting T (True), F (False) or D (Don't know) in the spaces provided.

1. A tremor of the outstretched hands
A is characteristic of Parkinson's disease
B responds to propranolol
C is often familial and benign
D may be worsened by anxiety
E is improved by primidone

Your answers: A.........B.........C.........D.........E.........

2. After a single seizure in adult life
A a patient is banned from driving for three years
B a normal EEG excludes epilepsy
C life long anticonvulsants should be started
D a patient may never hold a Heavy Goods Vehicle Licence
E a cerebral tumour is the most likely cause

Your answers: A.........B.........C.........D.........E.........

3. Extrapyramidal rigidity may be caused by
A butyrophenone tranquillisers
B B12 deficiency
C abuse of synthetic pethidine derivatives
D carbon monoxide poisoning
E the neuroleptic malignant syndrome

Your answers: A.........B.........C.........D.........E.........

Answers overleaf

ANSWERS AND EXPLANATIONS

1. **B C D E**

   The tremor of Parkinson's disease is characteristically a rest tremor, though a mild action tremor is sometimes seen. Action tremors like many tremors are worsened by anxiety. A marked action tremor may run in families and is seldom suggestive of serious neurological disease. Titubation of the head which is common in the elderly, is an action tremor of the neck muscles, is not a sign of Parkinson's disease and is usually benign. The drug of first choice for troublesome action tremors is propranolol but in patients in whom this drug is ineffective or contraindicated, low doses of primidone may be effective.

2. **D**

   A single seizure does not constitute epilepsy, for which label there should be more than one attack. However there is a 40-80% likelihood of further seizures most commonly within a year. An abnormal EEG increases the chance of further seizures as does a structural cause. If no EEG or structural abnormality is found further attacks may still occur and the patient should not drive for at least one year. If more than one attack occurs, driving is disallowed until two years have passed without seizures during wakefulness. If all seizures have occurred during sleep for a period of three years, driving is allowed even if sleep seizures continue. A Heavy Goods Licence is permanently disallowed for any seizure occurring after the age of five years. The commonest diagnosed cause of epilepsy in adult life is cerebrovascular disease (up to 50% in patients over 50 years). Anticonvulsants are not usually started after a single seizure unless there is good reason to suspect recurrence (see above).

3. **A C D E**

   Phenothiazine and butyrophenone tranquillisers block the D2 dopamine receptors in the corpus striatum and are the principal causes of iatrogenic Parkinsonism. In the early 1980s, a severe parkinsonian syndrome appeared in Californian drug addicts caused principally by 1-methyl-4-phenyl-1,2,5,6-tetrahydropyridine (MPTP), a by-product of synthetic opiate manufacture. The neuroleptic malignant syndrome is a rare, life threatening complication of neuroleptic therapy which may also follow withdrawal from amantidine. Features include hyperpyrexia, severe extrapyramidal rigidity and autonomic disturbances. Treatment is by withdrawal of the neuroleptic drug and administration of dantrolene and/or bromocriptine.

4. Selegiline is a newly developed
  A tranquilliser for use in major psychoses
  B monoamine oxidase B inhibitor
  C anti-parkinsonian agent
  D agent which increases the availability of dopamine to the nigro-striatal pathway
  E antidepressant

    Your answers: A.........B.........C.........D.........E.........

5. Focal delta (slow) wave activity on EEG
  A is a common normal finding in adults
  B indicates the presence of a focal structural lesion
  C indicates the need for further investigation
  D is found after a major cerebral infarction
  E indicates the presence of epilepsy

    Your answers: A.........B.........C.........D.........E.........

6. Dopa decarboxylase inhibitors
  A block the post-synaptic dopamine receptors in the substantia nigra
  B prevent the extra-cerebral complications of L-dopa therapy
  C increase the availability of dopamine to the corpus striatum
  D act in Parkinson's disease by inhibiting the oxidation of dopamine in the synaptic cleft
  E prevent L-dopa associated dyskinesias

    Your answers: A.........B.........C.........D.........E.........

Answers overleaf

4. **B C D**

Dopamine is metabolised by monoamine oxidase B. Selegiline inhibits this enzyme and therefore increases the availability of dopamine to the nigro-striatal pathway. Its use in the management of Parkinson's disease is still to be explored but its main usefulness is in smoothing out the response swings to L-dopa therapy seen later in the disease. If monoamine oxidase B is found to be related to the pathogenesis of the disease, there may be a role for the earlier use of this drug to prevent progression of the substantia nigra degeneration. Selegiline is not associated with toxic 'cheese' reactions caused by ingestion of foods high in tyramine. This may be because the facilitated noradrenaline released from its binding sites which causes the 'cheese' effect with the antidepressant monoamine oxidase inhibitors is distinct from monoamine oxidase B inhibition and selegiline does not act on the former receptors.

5. **B C D**

Focal delta wave activity, particularly if continuous, suggests the presence of a structural brain lesion, but is pathologically non-specific and may occur after substantial vascular lesions of any type, tumours or even advanced neurodegenerative disease. Neurophysiologically this abnormality represents an area of electrically inactive cortex which allows the appearance on the surface EEG of underlying slow waves probably originating from the thalamic rhythm generators. The appearance of focal delta wave activity is an indication for further investigation by CT scanning. Although seizures may occur with such structural lesions the EEG appearances are not synonymous with clinical seizures, focal slow waves being seen in many patients with comparable structural lesions who have not had seizures.

6. **B**

The dopa decarboxylase inhibitors, carbidopa and benserazide, inhibit the conversion of L-dopa to dopamine outside the central nervous system. This prevents the peripheral side-effects of L-dopa such as cardiac arrhythmias, hypotension, anorexia and vomiting. In addition there is probably a more reliable level of L-dopa and therefore dopamine achievable in the central nervous system, this may go some way to smooth out variability in response but does not prevent dyskinesias. It is the monoamine oxidase B inhibitors such as selegiline which inhibit the oxidation of dopamine and so increase the availability of dopamine to the striatum.

7. Optic neuritis

A is almost always followed by other symptoms of multiple sclerosis

B causes an ipsilateral increased latency of the visual evoked P100 potential

C indicates the presence of an ipsilateral carotid stenosis

D the presence of oligoclonal bands on CSF examination increases the probability of future attacks of central demyelination

E may be accompanied by an afferent pupillary defect

Your answers: A.........B.........C.........D.........E.........

8. Muscle fasciculations

A occur with reinnervation of partially denervated muscles

B in the calf muscles are often benign

C may be seen during an edrophonium test for myasthenia gravis

D are diagnostic of motor neurone disease

E occur in spinal muscular atrophy

Your answers: A.........B.........C.........D.........E.........

9. Myasthenia gravis

A is caused by autoantibodies directed against acetylcholine

B in older men responds to thymectomy, especially if a thymoma is present

C responds to high dose steroid therapy

D may be worsened by aminoglycoside antibiotics

E may be treated by long-term edrophonium therapy

Your answers: A.........B.........C.........D.........E.........

Answers overleaf

7. B D E

Optic neuritis presents with a subacute, usually unilateral visual loss which usually recovers over a period of some weeks. It should not be confused with the sudden transient unilateral visual loss (amaurosis fugax) caused by emboli from the ipsilateral carotid artery. In arteriopathic individuals subacute ischaemic optic neuropathy may present with subacute visual loss not caused by embolism. After an attack of optic neuritis the risk of multiple lesions varies between 35 and 75%. The presence of oligoclonal pattern on CSF electrophoresis and the presence of the HLA-DR2 tissue type antigen increase the likelihood of lesions in other parts of the nervous system.

8. A B C E

Fasciculations consist of spontaneous contractions of single motor units visible to the naked eye. They are frequently seen in the quadriceps and calf muscles of healthy individuals and by themselves are not diagnostic of MND. In the latter disease the fasciculations are seen in many more muscles and associated with wasting, weakness and other features of MND. Fasciculations may occur pathologically in many situations where there is partial denervation e.g. root lesions. The origin is probably in the electrical instability of the reinnervation (and excessive sensitivity to acetylcholine) that occurs in chronic partial denervation. Though not frequently seen in spinal muscular atrophy, fasciculations may occasionally be found in adult onset cases.

9. C D

The pathogenic mechanism in myasthenia gravis is the production of autoantibodies directed against the acetylcholine receptors on the motor end plate. These are present in 90% of patients with myasthenia although their titre correlates poorly with the clinical severity of the disease. Myasthenia in younger women is usually not associated with thymoma and responds well to thymectomy. Older men with myasthenia are most likely to have a thymoma: present in about 10% of patients. Thymectomy in patients with thymoma usually has a disappointing effect on the myasthenia. Aminoglycoside antibiotics can worsen neuromuscular transmission in patients with myasthenia and may provoke onset. Edrophonium is too short acting for therapeutic use and is reserved for diagnostic purposes only.

10. Demyelinating peripheral neuropathy
A causes increased latency of sensory action potentials
B produces motor conduction velocities in the region of 40 m/sec
C may be caused by diphtheria toxin
D is the abnormality in some with the Charcot-Marie-Tooth syndrome
E is a feature of infection with *Mycobacterium leprae*

Your answers: A.........B.........C.........D.........E.........

11. In a patient with diplopia
A the paretic eye carries the most peripheral of the two images
B retained capacity of the eye to intort indicates a superior oblique palsy
C if the eye is deviated down and out the third cranial nerve is involved
D failure of the eye to abduct indicates a fourth cranial nerve palsy
E the lateral rectus is weak if the adducted eye cannot be depressed

Your answers: A.........B.........C.........D.........E.........

12. Concentric needle EMG recording
A shows large wide multiphasic potentials in denervation
B is always abnormal in metabolic myopathies
C shows spontaneous muscle fibre activity in polymyositis
D can confirm the diagnosis of motor neurone disease
E can be diagnostic in myotonic dystrophy

Your answers: A.........B.........C.........D.........E.........

Answers overleaf

10. A C D E

The effect of demyelination on a peripheral nerve is to slow impulse conduction. In focal demyelination the local sensory action potential is delayed in latency and only somewhat decreased in amplitude. In more severe and diffuse demyelination the sensory action potentials may no longer be demonstrable. The neuropathy caused by the diphtheria toxin is due to an effect on Schwann cells inhibiting the maintenance of the myelin sheath. Charcot-Marie-Tooth syndrome is the clinical presentation of a number of congenital disorders including hereditary sensorimotor neuropathies of axonal and demyelinating type and late onset spinal muscular atrophy. The leprosy bacteria infect the Schwann cells of peripheral nerves near the skin surface, causing a multifocal demyelinating neuropathy.

11. A C

When assessing the cause of diplopia the first task is to determine which eye is involved. The cover test is the simplest method. When the paretic eye is covered, the most peripheral of the two images will disappear. The diplopia will be maximal in the direction of gaze produced by the paretic muscle. The main action of the superior oblique muscle is to depress the adducted eye. Adduction is not possible with a third nerve palsy and the eye is usually deviated down and out by the effect of the still intact lateral rectus and superior oblique. In a third nerve palsy, the action of the intact superior oblique can be seen by its secondary action of intorsion of the eye (watch a conjunctival blood vessel whilst the patient tries to look at the tip of his nose).

12. A C E

The sampling of a skeletal muscle with a concentric needle electrode allows recording of the action potential of the motor unit close to the needle tip. In chronic partial denervation (as in motor neurone disease) re-innervation of denervated motor units occurs by sprouting intact neurones. This results in the number of fibres in a unit being increased (increasing the amplitude of the action potential), an increase in the duration of the action potential and its dispersal in space (producing a multiphasic wide potential recorded from the needle). The other electrophysiological features of motor neurone disease are normal peripheral sensory and motor nerve conduction times. Polymyositis produces spontaneous potentials in recordings from resting muscle. In myotonic disorders the EMG records a characteristic crescendo of potentials which produces a loudspeaker noise like a dive-bomber.

13. Sarcoidosis in the nervous system
A may be present without other evidence of sarcoid
B can present with diabetes insipidus
C causes a CSF lymphocyte pleocytosis
D causes the appearance of oligoclonal bands in the CSF
E may present with an intracranial mass

Your answers: A.......B.........C.........D.........E.........

14. Vertical nystagmus
A if upbeating, may indicate cerebellar tonsillar ectopia
B may occur with phenytoin toxicity
C if downbeating, indicates a lesion at the foramen magnum
D when present in an unconscious patient indicates a thalamic lesion
E may present with the symptom of ocillopsia

Your answers: A.......B.........C.........D.........E.........

15. After a major cerebral infarction
A a CT scan usually shows a low attenuation area within 2 hours
B the unenhanced scan may be normal in the second week
C contrast enhancement on the CT scan is maximal in the second week
D a mass effect from ischaemic oedema is seen on the CT scan in the first 6 hours
E carotid arteriography may be normal

Your answers: A.......B.........C.........D.........E.........

Answers overleaf

13. **A B C D E**

The manifestations of sarcoidosis in the nervous system are protean and may occur in the absence of extraneural involvement. Granulomatous meningeal inflammation causes many of the manifestations, including multiple cranial nerve palsies and radiculopathies. Inflammation of the basal meninges may present as diabetes insipidus and or hydrocephalus. Isolated collections of granulomatous inflammation may present as intracranial masses. Other signs include peripheral neuropathy and myelopathy. The CSF is usually abnormal with an increase in the protein content which may show oligoclonal IgG bands often with an increased cell count.

14. **B C E**

Drug toxicity (for example with phenytoin) may cause nystagmus in all directions, horizontal and vertical. If the fast phase is downbeating the lesion is usually low in the medulla near the cervico-medullary junction. Masses at this site (or the congenital Arnold-Chiari malformation) may present with a combination of occipital pain, ataxia and downbeating nystagmus. There may or may not be an oscillopsia, a sensation of the visual field bouncing up and down with the nystagmus. Nystagmus does not occur in unconscious patients since the fast phase appears to depend on intact hemisphere function. In an unconscious patient with a thalamic lesion the eyes may be deviated downwards.

15. **B C E**

Up to the first 12 hours or so after even a substantial cerebral infarction the CT scan may show very little change. In fact the extent of the low attenuation area caused by an infarction usually does not become clear for at least 12 hours and sometimes longer. Over the first 24-36 hours the ischaemic tissue swells, producing a mass effect on the scan by the second or third day which then subsides by the first week. Towards the end of the first week the infarcted tissue is invaded by phagocytic glial cells which may increase the X-ray attenuation of the area so that the plain scan looks normal. However the infarct is also invaded by new blood vessels which show as areas of enhancement after injection of iodinated contrast medium. This post-contrast enhancement is maximal during the second week after the infarction. Carotid angiography after cerebral infarction may be normal even after substantial infarction. This occurs particularly following embolism when the causative occlusion may disperse. In such cases the longer after the stroke the angiogram is performed the more likely it is to be normal.

16. **Regular generalised 3 Hz spike and wave activity on EEG**
    A confirms the diagnosis of complex partial epilepsy
    B indicates the presence of a local structural lesion
    C is associated with transient 'absence' attacks in children
    D is seen during tonic-clonic seizures in adults
    E is a diagnostic feature of herpes encephalitis

    Your answers: A.......B.........C.........D.........E.........

17. **A macular sparing hemianopia**
    A indicates a lesion in the optic radiation
    B indicates a vascular lesion in the parietal lobe
    C does not prevent a patient from reading
    D will exclude a patient from holding a driving licence
    E suggests a lesion in the posterior cerebral artery territory

    Your answers: A.......B.........C.........D.........E.........

18. **In a young person with an internuclear ophthalmoplegia**
    A oligoclonal bands in the CSF confirm the diagnosis of multiple sclerosis
    B unilateral delay in the visual evoked potentials is strong evidence of the diagnosis of multiple sclerosis
    C indicates the presence of extrinsic brain stem compression
    D if demyelination is the cause, high doses of intravenous steroids will speed recovery
    E the lesion is in the median longitudinal fasciculus in the brainstem

    Your answers: A.........B.........C.........D.........E.........

Answers overleaf

16. **C**

The syndrome of frequent absence attacks combined with generalised 3 Hz spike and wave activity is known as petit mal epilepsy. This is a primary generalised epilepsy not associated with structural abnormalities. Localised structural lesions are often associated with either focal slow wave activity or a sharp wave focus. A complex partial seizure is one in which focal epileptic symptoms (often from the temporal lobe) are associated with impairment of awareness, during which time the patient is inaccessible. The EEG during tonic-clonic seizures in adults usually shows a combination of fast activity with large amplitude slow waves with or without polyspike or spike-wave activity. In herpes simplex encephalitis there is a focal abnormality in about 80% of cases. Typical changes are periodic slow waves and/or spikes from one or both temporal lobes.

17. **C D E**

The macular region of the visual cortex is at the tip of the occipital lobe on its medial aspect and is supplied with blood by both the middle and posterior cerebral arteries. The result is that an infarction in the posterior cerebral artery territory causes a homonymous hemianopia which spares the macular region. Patients can usually read with this deficit since the ability to scan is retained. Lesions which interrupt the optic radiation in the parietal lobe cause a hemianopia which involves the macula and there are often visuoperceptual deficits which interfere with the ability to read. A patient with a visual field defect below the horizon of vision is not permitted to hold a driving licence.

18. **B D E**

The diagnosis of multiple sclerosis depends on the demonstration of central nervous system lesions disseminated in time and place. An internuclear ophthalmoplegia is a sign of an intrinsic brainstem lesion affecting the median longitudinal fasciculus. If the spinal fluid is shown to contain gammaglobulin in an oligoclonal pattern multiple sclerosis is very likely. However oligoclonal bands are present in many other intrathecal inflammatory diseases and do not make multiple sclerosis certain. If a delayed visual evoked response is demonstrated in a patient with an internuclear ophthalmoplegia, multiple sclerosis is probable. If there is a past history of optic neuritis the diagnosis is confirmed. In multiple sclerosis, high dose intravenous steroids have been shown to shorten the duration of relapses though they probably have no effect on long-term disability.

19. In spasticity

A baclofen acts as a GABA-antagonist on spinal cord inter-neurones

B baclofen increases presynaptic inhibition of spinal motor-neurones

C baclofen may cause drowsiness in excessive dosage

D dantrolene sodium acts as a GABA-mimetic in the spinal cord

E calcium release inhibition in skeletal muscle is the mode of action of dantrolene sodium

Your answers: A.........B.........C.........D.........E.........

20. In the carpal tunnel syndrome

A there is increased latency of the median sensory action potential

B wasting of the whole of the thenar eminence occurs

C Tinel's sign is usually negative

D there is delay in the median distal motor latency

E in a severe case there will be weakness of extensor pollicis brevis

Your answers: A.........B.........C.........D.........E.........

21. Huntington's chorea

A is inherited as an autosomal recessive characteristic

B may present with extrapyramidal rigidity in younger victims

C always becomes clinically apparent by the third decade of life

D is associated with loss of volume of the caudate nucleus on CT scans

E usually responds to L-dopa therapy

Your answers: A.........B.........C.........D.........E.........

Answers overleaf

19. B C E

In spasticity there is relative underactivity of the spinal cord GABA interneurones which normally exert presynaptic inhibition of spinal motorneurones. Baclofen is a GABA-agonist which has a beneficial effect on spasticity but may cause drowsiness in excessive dosage. Furthermore sometimes the removal of spasticity may reveal that the limbs are weak and thus paradoxically worsen the patient's disability. Dantrolene is a drug acting against spasticity which works at a more peripheral level, probably by inhibiting sarcoplasmic calcium release, thus reducing muscle contractility.

20. A D

Tinel's sign is positive when tapping the wrist causes paraesthesia in the digits supplied by the median nerve and is a sign of the carpal tunnel syndrome. Only three of the muscles of the thenar eminence are supplied by the median nerve, the abductor pollicis brevis, opponens pollicis and the flexor pollicis brevis. Prolongation of the latency of the sensory action potential is electrophysiological evidence of median nerve compression at the wrist, with progressive reduction of its amplitude as denervation occurs. Similarly the distal motor latency to median supplied muscles (abductor pollicis brevis is usually tested) is delayed in the face of normal motor conduction proximal to the wrist.

21. B D

Huntington's chorea is inherited as an autosomal dominant characteristic with near complete penetrance. However the age of onset varies and may be delayed until the fifth or sixth decade of life. In younger patients there may be marked extrapyramidal rigidity, such juvenile onset cases having usually inherited the Huntington's gene from their father rather than their mother. The volume of caudate nucleus can be reduced on CT scan but this is not a reliable test particularly early in the course of the disorder. L-dopa will worsen the choreic movements of patients with Huntington's, the therapy for which is tetrabenazine. Major tranquillisers in the phenothiazine and butyrophenone classes may be necessary in more severely hyperkinetic patients.

22. After aneurysmal subarachnoid haemorrhage (SAH)

A the syndrome of inappropriate ADH secretion may occur

B the peak risk for secondary ischaemic complications is immediately after the haemorrhage

C the risk of rebleeding is maximal in the month following the stroke

D a catecholamine surge can cause direct myocardial damage

E if the patient is comatose, referral for early aneurysm clipping is generally advised

Your answers: A.........B.........C.........D.........E.........

23. In Bell's palsy

A the majority recover without residual weakness

B a complete facial weakness is a poor prognostic sign

C if the palsy is complete, tarsorrhaphy is usually required to protect the cornea

D mild sensory symptoms at onset are a common feature

E electrophysiological tests may be helpful prognostically

Your answers: A.........B.........C.........D.........E.........

24. Gait ataxia

A is a sign of a cerebellar hemisphere lesion

B may be the presenting features of benign intracranial hypertension

C is a presenting sign of cerebellar ectopia

D occurs as a feature of carbamazepine toxicity

E occurs in cerebellar vermis lesions

Your answers: A.........B.........C.........D.........E.........

Answers overleaf

22. A C D

Hypothalamic damage frequently occurs after substantial SAH due to berry aneurysms. This causes excessive ADH secretion and is probably the cause of the surge of catecholamines which may cause life-threatening cardiac arrhythmias and subendocardial myocardial necrosis. There is usually a delay of some days (with a peak incidence in the second week) after SAH before secondary ischaemic changes become apparent. The risk of rebleeding, compared with deterioration due to vasospasm, has probably been overestimated and falls fairly sharply from up to 50% within the first month (in unoperated patients) such that at six months it is 3% per year. In general neurosurgeons do not consider aneurysmal clipping in patients who are unconscious since the outlook for such patients is so poor. Referral for such surgery is therefore delayed until the clinical condition of the patient has improved (provided that the diagnosis is clear).

23. A B D E

The unilateral lower motor neurone palsy of unknown origin known as Bell's palsy is often preceded by pain in the mastoid region. At least 80% of cases show complete recovery but total paralysis at onset is a poor prognostic sign. In the latter case recovery does occur but cross reinnervation may produce unsatisfactory results. Tarsorrhaphy to protect the cornea is hardly ever necessary in Bell's palsy, though a supply of artificial tears (hydroxymellose drops) may be necessary. Corneal sensation is always intact and the uprolling of the eye to blink (the Bell's phenomenon) is usually sufficient protection of the cornea before spontaneous recovery occurs. After about three weeks, if recovery has not occurred EMG tests may help predict prognosis. If there is no evidence of denervation the prognosis for recovery is good.

24. C D E

Lesions in one or other cerebellar hemisphere usually cause peripheral limb ataxia (e.g. 'finger to nose ataxia') rather than ataxia of gait which is a feature of central cerebellar (vermis) lesions. Gait ataxia is associated with normal pressure hydrocephalus not benign intracranial hypertension. Cerebellar ectopia may present with a combination of gait ataxia and nystagmus (often downbeating vertically). Gait ataxia and other cerebellar signs are features of alcohol and anticonvulsant (including carbamazepine) toxicity.

25. Benign intracranial hypertension (BIH)
A may present with transient visual obscurations
B is a complication of anorexia nervosa
C is associated with enlarged cerebral ventricles on CT scan
D may complicate vitamin D toxicity
E is treated by repeated lumbar puncture

Your answers: A.........B.........C.........D.........E.........

26. In neurosyphilis
A a normal CSF excludes active disease
B syphilitic serology may be positive in the CSF when negative in the serum
C oligoclonal bands in the CSF indicate active disease
D the pupils are small and unreactive to accommodation
E dementia may be a presenting feature

Your answers: A.........B.........C.........D.........E.........

27. Chronic subdural haematomas (CSH)
A commonly present without a history of recent cranial trauma
B may present with acute stroke-like episodes with a clear conscious level
C are seen on CT scan as high density lesions
D may not be visible on an unenhanced CT scan
E always require surgical evacuation

Your answers: A.........B.........C.........D.........E.........

Answers overleaf

25. A E

Despite raised pressure causing papilloedema BIH is a syndrome in which consciousness is clear and there are no focal neurological signs (although false localising signs such as sixth nerve palsies may occur). It may present with headache and transient visual obscurations which forewarn of visual failure. The cerebral ventricles are normal or smaller than usual, i.e. hydrocephalus is not present. BIH is not a feature of anorexia nervosa but occurs in young obese females often with menstrual irregularities. Other causes include pregnancy, the contraceptive pill, hypocortisolism, hypoparathyroidism, hyper and hypovitaminosis A, tetracycline therapy and other drugs. Usually BIH is a self-limiting condition but because of the risk of visual loss, treatment with repeated lumbar puncture is advised. Steroids and carbonic anhydrase inhibitors have been suggested but are not usually effective.

26. A C E

Neurosyphilis may present with dementia and few other signs. In active CNS infection with *Treponema pallidum* the CSF shows an increase in cells and protein. The serological tests for syphilis may remain positive in the CSF long after the CNS infection becomes inactive. The serum tests for syphilis are usually positive when the CNS is infected and blood tests (e.g. VDRL and TPHA) are an adequate screen for neurosyphilis. In the presence of active infection oligoclonal bands of IgG may be identified. The Argyl-Robertson pupils of classic syphilitic infection are small, irregular and though reacting to accommodation do not constrict to light.

27. A D

A history of head injury is not obtained in up to half of the patients with CSH. Although patients with CSH may present with acute focal signs, when this occurs the level of consciousness is always altered, usually in a fluctuant manner. If the subdural haematoma is chronic it will show as a low density area on the CT scan rather than the high density area which characterises acute subdural collections of blood. In an intermediate phase the collection may be the same density as brain and therefore, particularly if bilateral, missed on plain scans. If however, such an isodense subdural is unilateral it may still be detected on the scan by the shift it causes in the intracranial contents. Some subdural haematomas are not evacuated if, by the time they are discovered, the level of consciousness is unaltered and there is little shift on the scan. However follow-up CT scans are mandatory.

28. Myoclonus
A is a sign seen in metabolic encephalopathy
B is a feature of the Gilles de la Tourette syndrome
C with dementia is a feature of Jacob-Creutzfeldt disease
D may occur with childhood epilepsy
E is a feature of chronic anoxic encephalopathy

Your answers: A.........B.........C.........D.........E.........

29. In motor neurone disease (MND)
A sensory symptoms at onset do not exclude the diagnosis
B peripheral motor conduction velocities are normal
C the function of the glossopharyngeal nerve is frequently affected
D the onset of bulbar palsy indicates a poor prognosis
E the abdominal reflexes are usually preserved

Your answers: A.........B.........C.........D.........E.........

30. Oligodendroglioma of the nervous system
A are derived from cells of the lymphocyte series
B occur with increased frequency in immunosuppressed patients
C are slow growing tumours associated with long survival following diagnosis
D often show calcification on CT scanning
E are derived from the myelin producing cells of the central nervous system

Your answers: A.........B.........C.........D.........E.........

Answers overleaf

28. **A C D E**

Myoclonus consists of quick muscle jerks which may be sporadic or rhythmic and may be sparked off by attempts at voluntary movements. Myoclonus may be associated with epilepsy, particularly in childhood and various other disorders including acute metabolic encephalopathies (e.g. renal and hepatic failure). Jacob-Creutzfeldt disease is a slow virus infection which causes a subacute spongiform encephalopathy, presenting with a rapidly progressive dementia with myoclonus. Severe action myoclonus may also follow recovery from global anoxia such as after prolonged cardiac arrest. The Gilles de la Tourette syndrome is a syndrome of multiple tics and involuntary vocalisations in which myoclonus is not a feature. Tics are semi-purposeful and can be suppressed to some degree, unlike myoclonus which is completely involuntary and random.

29. **A B D E**

Some patients have vague sensory symptoms in the early stages of MND and limb pain is a surprisingly frequent problem later in the disease. However sensory *signs* are never present. Essential to the diagnosis is the demonstration that the peripheral motor and sensory conduction times are normal. The glossopharyngeal nerve is purely sensory and so is not affected in MND, thus severe bulbar problems may be present, but palatal sensation is normal. The prognosis for life in MND once bulbar symptoms develop is usually measured in months. The abdominal reflexes, which usually disappear in the face of upper motor neurone lesions, are often strangely preserved in MND, the explanation is unknown.

30. **C D E**

Oligodendroglial cells are the central nervous system equivalent to the Schwann cell in that they synthesise myelin and perform various nutritive and supporting roles for the central neurones. By contrast microglial cells are the CNS equivalent of lymphocytes, and tumours of this series of cells are more frequent in immunosuppressed patients. Oligodendrogliomas are often slow growing although they may show more malignant transformation after some years. This slow growth is reflected in the frequent finding of calcification visible on CT scans. The tumours frequently present with epilepsy rather than focal signs or raised intracranial pressure.

31. Neurofibromatosis

A may be complicated by carotid artery occlusion

B is associated with an increased incidence of cerebral microgliomas

C is suggested by the presence of more than five café-au-lait spots

D may be complicated by bilateral sensorineural deafness

E is inherited as an autosomal dominant characteristic

Your answers: A.........B.........C.........D.........E.........

32. Metachromatic leucodystrophy

A may present in infancy with a peripheral neuropathy

B is caused by a deficiency of hexosaminidase A enzyme

C is a cause of dementia in young adults

D is always associated with an elevated CSF protein concentration in adult-onset cases

E in adults is associated with low density white matter on CT scanning

Your answers: A.........B.........C.........D.........E.........

33. Infarction in the territory of the anterior cerebral artery

A causes more severe hand than shoulder weakness on the affected side

B produces predominant weakness of the lower limb

C is most frequently seen after subarachnoid haemorrhage due to berry aneurysm rupture

D causes transcortical motor aphasia when affecting the dominant hemisphere

E usually occurs as a result of cerebral embolism

Your answers: A.........B.........C.........D.........E.........

Answers overleaf

31. A C D E

Neurofibromatosis is the commonest autosomal dominantly inherited neurocutaneous disorder. The hallmark of the disease is a combination of multiple pigmented 'café-au-lait' spots, cutaneous neurofibromas and plexiform neuromas. There is a tendency to develop schwannomas and neurofibromas on peripheral and cranial nerves. There may be bilateral acoustic neuromas and a tendency to develop cerebral astrocytomas, particularly optic gliomas. In children cerebrovascular occlusive disease including carotid occlusion may occur. More than five 'café-au-lait' spots measuring 1.5 cm or more are suggestive of the diagnosis and axillary freckling is a characteristic feature. Further complications include phaeochromocytoma, Wilms' tumour and non-lymphocytic leukaemia.

32. A C E

Metachromatic leucodystrophy is one of the commonest congenital storage diseases of the nervous system, due to defective synthesis of the enzyme arylsulphatase A. In infancy and childhood metachromatic leucodystrophy presents with intellectual impairment, gait disorder, spasticity, optic atrophy and peripheral neuropathy. In adult onset cases the presentation is usually with dementia or psychoses with or without a peripheral neuropathy. The CSF protein content is often though not invariably elevated. CT scanning may show widespread low densities in the cerebral white matter. The defective arylsulphatase A leads to an accumulation of sulphatides in the urine.

33. B C D

Anterior cerebral artery territory infarction is almost always caused by secondary vasospasm following subarachnoid haemorrhage. Infarction in this territory causes predominant weakness of the lower limb and the proximal upper limb (the shoulder). The hand may be weakened by damage to the underlying fibres of the internal capsule but is less severely affected. If the dominant hemisphere is damaged there is a non-fluent aphasia (reduced word output) with good understanding and preserved ability to repeat words (transcortical motor aphasia). Damage to the anterior cerebral artery territory due to cerebral embolism is almost unheard of.

34. In an unconscious patient
A the presence of a flexion withdrawal response in the limbs excludes brain death
B drug overdose may reproduce all the clinical signs of brain death
C nystagmus on cold water irrigation of the ears indicates that the patient is feigning coma
D large, minimally reactive pupils indicate a pontine lesion
E medium sized irregular pupils indicate a thalamic lesion

Your answers: A.........B.........C.........D.........E.........

35. The following are associated with peripheral neuropathy:
A thallium poisoning
B tetracycline therapy
C anti-tuberculous therapy
D scarlet fever
E carcinoma of the bronchus

Your answers: A.........B.........C.........D.........E.........

36. Spinal muscular atrophy (SMA)
A may present in adult life with distal muscle wasting
B is characterised by a combination of upper and lower motor neurone signs
C is characterised by EMG evidence of chronic partial denervation
D does not cause pseudobulbar palsy
E is a primary disorder of anterior horn cells

Your answers: A.........B.........C.........D.........E.........

Answers overleaf

34. B C E

In a patient who is brain dead, painful stimuli to the limbs may cause slight flexion withdrawal which is a spinal reflex and does not indicate residual brainstem or cerebral function. Whilst drug overdose can mimic all the signs of brain death, the criteria for the diagnosis of death require that the cause of the coma be known and that drug overdose (and hypothermia) are specifically excluded. Nystagmus does not occur in genuinely unconscious patients. Pontine lesions are usually associated with extremely small, minimally responsive pupils. Thalamic lesions causing coma often produce medium sized, sometimes eccentric pupils with little reaction to light.

35. A C E

Thallium salts, which are used as pesticides, cause a predominantly motor neuropathy of acute onset which may be confused with the Guillain-Barré syndrome. Hair loss is a later feature of thallium poisoning and may be a diagnostic clue. Antibacterial drugs which may cause a peripheral neuropathy include nitrofurantoin, ethambutol and isoniazid. The latter occurs in slow acetylators of the drug and may be prevented by pyridoxine therapy. Carcinoma of the lung may be associated with a paraneoplastic sensorimotor neuropathy and occasionally a pure sensory neuropathy, though the latter is more frequent with breast carcinoma.

36. A C D E

SMA are a group of inherited disorders of the lower motor neurone which may present in childhood or in adult life. Some varieties such as the autosomal recessive Werdnig-Hoffman disease may present with floppiness in infancy. Juvenile-onset SMA (Kugelberg-Weilander disease) is the commonest variety, presenting at ages 3-18 years with rather more slowly progressive muscular wasting later in childhood. Adult forms may present with Charcot-Marie-Tooth disease and less common varieties such as the X-linked recessive bulbospinal muscular atrophy may cause bulbar symptoms. Upper motor signs do not occur. The EMG shows chronic denervation with normal distal conduction times, which allows differentiation from muscular dystrophy or inherited peripheral neuropathy.

37. After intervertebral disc prolapse

A sensory loss is accompanied by reduced sensory action potentials in the relevant root distribution

B pain is felt in the muscles innervated by the damaged nerve root

C in the lumbar region may be accompanied by an extensor plantar response

D in the lumbar region loss of bladder function may result

E loss of the ankle reflex indicates an S1 root lesion

Your answers: A.........B.........C.........D.........E.........

38. In the Guillain-Barré syndrome

A sensory symptoms in the digits are a frequent early feature

B the CSF cell count is frequently elevated in the first few days of the illness

C the peak flow rate is the clearest guide to the need for artificial ventilation

D limb ataxia frequently occurs in severely affected patients

E there may be an underlying lymphoma

Your answers: A.........B.........C.........D.........E.........

39. Calcified cerebral lesions on a CT scan

A may be due to cerebral cysticercosis

B occur with metastatic colonic carcinoma

C if restricted to the basal ganglia may be found in normal people

D occur following herpes simplex encephalitis

E may follow cerebral malaria

Your answers: A.........B.........C.........D.........E.........

Answers overleaf

37. B D E

The dorsal root ganglia of the spinal roots are in the exit foramina of the spine. Compression by an intervertebral disc usually occurs proximal to this site and therefore the sensory action potential in the distal neurone is intact. Nerve root compression often causes pain which is felt in the muscles supplied by that segment, for example in the pectoralis muscle and triceps in a C7 root compression. Compression in the lumbar region cannot cause upper motor signs since the spinal cord ends at L1. A large central disc in the lower lumbar region may compress the sacral roots in the cauda equina and cause bladder symptoms. The root innervation of the ankle reflex is S1 so compression of this root will cause loss of the ankle jerk.

38. A B D E

Post-infective polyradiculopathy or the Guillain-Barré syndrome usually presents with sensory symptoms in the limbs followed by an ascending sensorimotor deficit. Severely affected cases show quite marked ataxia which cannot be entirely explained by joint-position loss and may be related to defective functioning of muscle spindle afferents. In the initial few days of symptoms the CSF cell count may be raised but later the classical pattern appears of high protein with a normal cell count. Since ventilation may be impaired in severe cases in which the bulbar musculature is denervated it is essential to monitor this. The test to use is the vital capacity, not the peak flow which is mainly a measure of airway size rather than ventilation volume. Uncommonly the Guillain-Barré syndrome may be the presenting feature of an underlying lymphoma.

39. A B C

In some parts of the world cysticercosis is the commonest cause of calcified intracerebral lesions. The presence of calcification often indicates that the infection with the pork tapeworm larva is no longer active. Metastases from the colon are another cause of multiple intracranial calcified lesions. Calcification in the basal ganglia may be a normal finding in some patients but also occurs in idiopathic hypoparathyroidism and pseudohypoparathyroidism. Herpes simplex encephalitis may leave scars of low density on CT scans but these do not calcify.

40. In a right sided hypoglossal nerve palsy
A the protruded tongue will deviate towards the left
B the soft palate will deviate towards the right
C if the neighbouring three cranial nerves are involved, the lesion is likely to be in the region of the jugular foramen
D taste will be impaired over the anterior two thirds of the tongue
E sensation will be impaired over the right side of the soft palate.

Your answers: A.........B.........C.........D.........E.........

41. Anterior spinal artery territory thrombosis
A causes loss of joint position in the limbs below the lesion
B rarely causes loss of bladder function
C will produce wasting of the intrinsic hand muscles if the lesion is at the C8/T1 level
D occurs following dissection of the thoracic aorta
E causes paraplegia with sparing of proprioception

Your answers: A.........B.........C.........D.........E.........

42. Infection with the human immunodeficiency virus (HIV)
A may present with an acute encephalopathy
B is a cause of epilepsy in adult life
C is a cause of primary dementia in young adults
D causes a peripheral neuropathy
E may present with a progressive spinal cord lesion

Your answers: A.........B.........C.........D.........E.........

Answers overleaf

Answers and Explanations

40. C

The twelfth cranial nerve or hypoglossal nerve innervates the musculature of the tongue. Paralysis of this musculature on one side causes the protruded tongue to be pushed over towards the weak side. The soft palate obtains its sensory innervation from the ninth (glossopharyngeal) cranial nerve and its motor innervation from the (tenth nerve) vagus. A combination of lesions on one side of cranial nerves 9, 10, 11 and 12 suggests that the lesion is at the jugular foramen just outside the skull, for example a glomus tumour. Taste over the anterior two thirds of the tongue is supplied by fibres which run in the facial nerve.

41. C D E

The anterior spinal artery supplies the anterior two thirds of the spinal cord with blood. In a dissection of the thoracic aorta loss of the blood flow to the anterior spinal artery from branches from the thoracic aorta may cause spinal infarction. The borderzone between the cord supply descending from the vertebral arteries and ascending from aortic branches is at the C8/T1 level and this may bear the brunt of the ischaemic insult. In this case there will be a lower motor neurone deficit at this segment causing intrinsic hand muscle wasting with a spastic paraparesis with bladder involvement but sparing of the dorsal columns and hence proprioception.

42. A B C D E

Infection with the HIV virus has sometimes been observed to cause an acute encephalopathy at the time of seroconversion. One of the commonest neurological manifestations of the acquired immunodeficiency syndrome caused by the HIV virus is cerebral toxoplasmosis which often presents with seizures, usually focal. There is growing evidence that the HIV virus is primarily neurotrophic and this may cause a dementia in long standing harbourers of the virus. Other neurological manifestations include a vacuolar myelopathy and a peripheral neuropathy.

43. **Binswanger's encephalopathy**
A is caused by organic mercurial poisoning
B may occur after global cerebral hypoperfusion
C is caused by small vessel cerebrovascular disease
D is identified on CT scan by multiple high density lesions
E is a cause of dementia in the elderly

Your answers: A.........B.........C.........D.........E.........

44. **The Eaton-Lambert syndrome**
A presents as fatiguable muscle weakness
B the muscle weakness responds to edrophonium injection
C the tendon reflexes are depressed
D the lesion is one of sarcoplasmic calcium transport
E is almost always associated with an underlying malignant neoplasm

Your answers: A.........B.........C.........D.........E.........

45. **The following disorders may present as the 'floppy infant syndrome':**
A Werdnig-Hoffman disease
B acid maltase deficiency
C Becker's muscular dystrophy
D myotonia congenita
E Kugelberg-Weilander disease

Your answers: A.........B.........C.........D.........E.........

43. B C E

Organic mercury poisoning causes a particular syndrome of cerebellar ataxia, paraesthesiae around the mouth and in the limbs, and concentric constriction of the visual fields. Binswanger's encephalopathy can now be recognised in life on CT scans as symmetrical low densities in the periventricular white matter with or without lacunar infarctions. Many patients with this manifestation of multiple small vessel ischaemic lesions are hypertensive. Similar CT and pathological lesions have been described following global hypoperfusion and in older patients with cerebral amyloid angiopathy. This subcortical ischaemic encephalopathy is a not infrequent cause of dementia in the elderly.

44. A B C

The myasthenic or Eaton-Lambert syndrome presents with fatiguable limb weakness usually without ptosis or bulbar symptoms. Autonomic features are common including a dry mouth, impotence and sphincter disturbances. In severe cases the weakness may be extensive and usually maximal proximally. Tendon reflexes are depressed or absent but increased by a period of muscle contraction (post-tetanic potentiation). The muscle weakness often responds to edrophonium but typically less so than in myasthenia gravis. In about one third of cases the Eaton- Lambert syndrome is not associated with underlying malignant disease. In this syndrome there is a decrease in the nerve evoked quantal release of acetylcholine, which is now thought to be due to antibodies directed against the calcium channel at the motor nerve terminal which results in inhibition of the release of acetylcholine from the terminal.

45. A B

Werdnig-Hoffman disease is the severest form of the congenital motor neurone diseases or spinal muscular atrophies and often presents as the 'floppy infant syndrome'. The Kugelberg-Weilander form of spinal muscular atrophy usually presents later in childhood. The infantile form of acid maltase deficiency presents as a floppy infant with cardiomegaly, enlargement of the liver and tongue followed by death usually before the age of two. Adult forms of the disease present in the second and third decades with a limb girdle pattern of muscular weakness. Myotonia congenita may present in infancy but causes myotonia with little weakness and progressive muscular hypertrophy. The myotonia is worse in the cold and accentuated by rest, so that the children have to 'warm up' before exercise.

46. The following are features of tuberose sclerosis
   A café-au-lait patches of pigmentation
   B ocular telangiectasias
   C cardiac rhabdomyomas
   D cerebral gliomas
   E cerebral aqueduct stenosis

   Your answers: A.........B.........C.........D.........E.........

47. Infantile spasms
   A present as generalised tonic-clonic seizures in early child-
   hood
   B are associated with three per second spike and wave acti-
   vity on EEG
   C occur in the first year of life
   D may be the presenting features of tuberose sclerosis
   E progress to other types of seizure in later life

   Your answers: A.........B.........C.........D.........E.........

48. Normal pressure hydrocephalus (NPH)
   A commonly presents with papilloedema with no focal signs
   B is characterised by the early onset of urinary incontinence
   C characteristically presents with dementia and gait distur-
   bance
   D is demonstrable on CT scan by hydrocephalus with a nor-
   mal sized fourth ventricle
   E may be improved by ventricular shunting

   Your answers: A.........B.........C.........D.........E.........

Answers overleaf

46. A C D

The classical lesions of tuberose sclerosis are adenoma sebaceum, red- brown papules in the butterfly distribution of the face, 'ash leaf' hypopigmented patches, and 'shagreen patches', usually over the lumbosacral area. However about 10% of patients have café-au-lait patches of pigmentation. Other CNS manifestations include epilepsy in association with cerebral malformations known as tubers and mental retardation. About 5% of children with tuberose sclerosis develop cerebral gliomas. Renal malformations may occur and cardiac rhabdomyomas are present in up to one third of patients.

47. C D E

Infantile spasms are sudden brief seizures consisting of jerks of one or more muscle groups, often presenting with sudden flexion spasms of the trunk (salaam spasm), presenting in the first year of life. There is often (but not always) an associated severe abnormality of the EEG known as 'hypsarrhythmia', consisting of high voltage random slow waves and spikes throughout the cortex. About one third of cases have no discoverable cause but in others there is a severe abnormality such as tuberose sclerosis, developmental anomalies, anoxia, infections and metabolic abnormalities. In about 50% of cases other types of seizures develop later in life including tonic-clonic seizures.

48. B C E

The classic clinical triad of NPH is dementia with early urinary incontinence and gait disturbance. Patients with NPH may not have these features but the CT scan appearance is often helpful since hydrocephalus is present with an enlarged fourth ventricle but normal or compressed cortical sulci (i.e. the pattern of communicating hydrocephalus). Many patients improve with ventricular shunting though prior CSF flow studies may be necessary to identify patients most likely to improve. If hydrocephalus is present with a normal sized fourth ventricle then the diagnosis is likely to be aqueduct stenosis or other obstructive lesion between the fourth and third ventricle. Papilloedema is not a feature of NPH.

49. In a spinal cord lesion

A hip flexion weakness is greater than hip extension weakness

B early bladder involvement suggests an intrinsic lesion

C Lhermitte's symptom suggests a thoracic cord lesion

D weakness of shoulder elevation suggests a lower cervical cord lesion

E intrinsic hand muscle wasting suggests a lesion above the C7 segment

Your answers: A.........B.........C.........D.........E.........

50. In Horner's syndrome

A the pupil on the affected side will dilate to hydroxy-amphetamine drops if the lesion is distal to the cervical ganglion

B occurs in the lateral medullary syndrome

C the affected pupil dilates more widely than the normal one with phenylephrine drops if the lesion is preganglionic

D the affected pupil fails to dilate with cocaine drops

E may be associated with injury to the upper trunks of the brachial plexus

Your answers: A.........B.........C.........D.........E.........

Answers overleaf

49. A B

The pattern of deficit seen in upper motor neurone lesions is for greatest weakness in the flexors of the lower limb and the extensors in the upper limb. On occasions this may be the only clue as to the site of the lesion. In compressive lesions bladder involvement usually occurs fairly late in the cord syndrome. By contrast intrinsic disorders such as demyelination often cause early urinary symptoms. In the presence of a cervical cord lesion (usually demyelination) flexion of the neck may cause paraesthesiae in the limbs. This is Lhermitte's symptom which may also occur with compressive lesions in the neck. The trapeziei, the main elevators of the shoulders are innervated by the spinal accessory nerve and their involvement suggests a very high cervical cord or medullary lesion. The intrinsic hand muscles are innervated by the first thoracic segment so wasting in these muscles in the presence of limb signs of a cord lesion indicates that the lesion is at T1.

50. B D

Horner's syndrome consists of mild ptosis, meiosis and variable loss of sweating over the affected side of the face. The lesion may be central, preganglionic or postganglionic according to its site with respect to the superior cervical ganglion. Hydroxyamphetamine drops release noradrenaline from the terminal axon if this is functioning and therefore dilate the pupil of central or preganglionic Horner's but not a postganglionic Horner's (because the axon is no longer functioning). Phenylephrine dilates the normal and abnormal pupil equally in both central and preganglionic peripheral type of Horner's. However in postganglionic Horner's denervation hypersensitivity causes the affected pupil to dilate more widely than the normal side. Cocaine blocks the re-uptake of noradrenaline from the neuromuscularjunction of the dilator muscle of the pupil, dilating the normal pupil. In any type of Horner's cocaine drops will not dilate the pupil of the affected eye, because noradrenaline is not being liberated into the nerve-muscle junction. The outflow of sympathetic innervation to the pupils is at T1 level and therefore Horner's syndrome may follow damage to the lower trunks of the brachial plexus.

Indicate your answers by putting T (True), F (False) or D (Don't know) in the spaces provided.

51. Schizophrenia
A occurs in 10% of the population
B is easily defined by careful mental state examination
C usually begins in the middle years of life
D is commoner in the United States than in Britain
E is extremely rare in patients with epilepsy

Your answers: A.........B.........C.........D.........E.........

52. Fragile-X syndrome is associated with the following features
A autosomal dominant inheritance
B male predominance
C bat ears
D the possibility of antenatal detection
E hyperkinetic syndrome

Your answers: A.........B.........C.........D.........E.........

53. Typical features of obsessive-compulsive neurosis include
A ruminations
B family history of neurosis
C rituals
D progression to schizophrenia
E resistance

Your answers: A.........B.........C.........D.........E.........

Answers overleaf

ANSWERS AND EXPLANATIONS

51. None are correct

Schizophrenia affects just under 1% of the population and usually begins in the third or fourth decade of life. Higher recorded rates in the United States than in Britain have been shown by crossnational research to reflect different diagnostic practices rather than a real difference in incidence. Thus, although assumed to reflect one or more underlying biological processes, schizophrenia is still in practice an arbitrarily defined concept. Although electroconvulsive treatment (ECT) was first introduced because epilepsy and schizophrenia were thought to be mutually exclusive, we now know schizophrenia-like psychoses are more common in epileptics than in the general population.

52. B C D E

Fragile-X syndrome has been recognised in recent years as the commonest cause of X-linked mental retardation. The cardinal features are male sex, facial abnormalities (bat ears, large jaw, maxillary hypoplasia) macro-orchidism and a marker (an apparent gap in the long arm of the X-chromosome) in lymphocytic culture under reducing conditions. This marker can be seen in amniotic fluid cells and therefore pre-natal diagnosis is possible. Carrier females are usually of normal intelligence, but about 10% have mild mental retardation. Recent reports have suggested high rates of infantile autism and hyperkinetic syndrome.

53. A C E

The key feature of an obsessional symptom is that the patient feels compelled to think or act in a certain way (compulsion) he recognises as absurd and attempts to resist (resistance). Ruminations are repetitive internal arguments about simple actions. Rituals are repeated irrational patterns of behaviour. There is probably a hereditary component in the aetiology of the condition but this is probably very small. The superficial similarity of obsessional symptoms and some of the features of schizophrenia is deceptive: there is no association between these two conditions.

54. In systemic lupus erythematosus (SLE)

A cerebral manifestations occur in less than 10% of cases
B schizophreniform psychosis is the commonest psychiatric manifestation
C psychiatric symptoms are almost always due to cerebral arteritis
D psychiatric symptoms usually precede fever and arthralgia
E cerebral involvement is an indicator of poor prognosis

Your answers: A.........B.........C.........D.........E.........

55. The following statements about alcohol dependence are true:

A withdrawal symptoms typically occur in the morning
B the commonest withdrawal symptoms are perceptual disturbances
C most alcohol-dependent patients develop liver cirrhosis
D intensive counselling has a significant effect on outcome
E chlormethiazole deters impulsive drinking via the acetaldehyde reaction

Your answers: A.........B.........C.........D.........E.........

56. After head injury there is an increased rate of

A depression
B schizophrenia
C dementia
D personality disorder
E suicide

Your answers: A.........B.........C.........D.........E.........

Answers overleaf

54. E

CNS involvement occurs in about one third of cases of SLE. Psychiatric symptoms occur in 60% of cases: the excess is due to both psychological reactions to illness and corticosteroid side effects. The commonest presentations are acute organic states and neurotic disorders; schizophrenia-like syndromes are rare. Mental symptoms are seldom the first signs of SLE (which are usually fever, malaise and arthralgia). When present, psychiatric symptoms often fluctuate, usually remit within six weeks but may recur. The presence of cerebral vasculitis substantially worsens prognosis.

55. A

Dependent alcoholics suffer withdrawal symptoms as their blood alcohol level falls. The commonest feature is acute tremulousness in the morning, often with agitation, nausea, retching and sweating. These and more severe features such as fleeting hallucinations, fits and clouding of consciousness can be reduced by inpatient detoxification with chlormethiazole or benzodiazepine cover. Disulfiram (Antabuse) is used as an aid to willpower as it blocks oxidation of alcohol and produces unpleasant flushing, nausea and headache. Liver cirrhosis occurs in 10% of alcoholics. Intensive programmes of counselling are probably no more effective than brief advice.

56. A B C D E

The most frequent sequelae of head injuries are minor neurotic symptoms, depression, fatigue, irritability and hypochondriasis, which occur even when there is no brain damage. Personality change, reduced drive, aggression, occurs notably after frontal lobe damage. Both depressive and schizophrenia-like psychoses are more frequent than in the general population. Lasting cognitive impairment is particularly associated with left temporal or parietal damage. The reason for the increased suicide rate is unclear.

57. The following statements about dementia are true:

A in most cases there is post mortem evidence of neurofibrillary tangles

B most affected patients reside in hospitals or residential homes

C an 85-year-old woman has a 20% risk of suffering from dementia

D loss of cholinergic activity correlates well with severity of symptoms in Alzheimer's-type dementia

E Pick's disease is probably caused by a 'slow virus'

Your answers: A.........B.........C.........D.........E.........

58. Recognised causes of depression include

A hyperthyroidism

B hyperparathyroidism

C L-tryptophan

D diazepam

E methyldopa

Your answers: A.........B.........C.........D.........E.........

59. Agoraphobic patients

A are usually female

B often have a fear of fainting

C benefit from aversion therapy

D usually have marital problems

E may report depersonalisation

Your answers: A.........B.........C.........D.........E.........

Answers overleaf

57. A C D

Dementia increases in incidence with age, at its peak affecting 20% of people in their ninth decade. The commonest form is Alzheimer's disease, pathologically defined by widespread senile plaques and neurofibrillary tangles. Reduction in biochemical markers of the cholinergic system are proportional to cognitive deficits. Pick's disease is a rare pre-senile dementia affecting frontal and temporal lobes. Creutzfeld-Jakob disease is transmitted by a 'slow virus'. At all ages, the great majority of demented patients live at home.

58. A B D E

Most cases of depression have no organic cause, but a wide variety of medical conditions and medications can produce depression. These include electrolyte disturbances (especially potassium depletion, hypocalcaemia and hypercalcaemia), endocrine disorders (Cushing's, Addison's, thyrotoxicosis, myxoedema and diabetes), other medical disorders (carcinoma, SLE, infections and neurological disease) and drugs (e.g. reserpine, L-dopa, methyldopa, betablockers and benzodiazepines). L-tryptophan is a precursor of serotonin and is used as adjunctive therapy for depression.

59. A B E

The symptoms of agoraphobia include physical symptoms of anxiety; depersonalisation (a subjective feeling that one's body is unreal or remote); thoughts focussed on fear of losing control, falling or fainting, and avoidance of certain situations notably crowds, shops and transport. Affected patients are predominantly female. Although they often become highly dependent on their husbands, the rate of marital conflict is not increased. Aversion therapy is used to extinguish unwanted behaviour. In agoraphobia, the aim is to encourage certain behaviours in controlled conditions; the preferred behavioural treatment is programmed practice.

60. The following statements about mental retardation are true:

A in mild retardation, subcultural influences are pre-eminent

B there is an increased risk of psychosis

C treatment for phenylketonuria should be continued for life

D the features of cretinism are present at birth

E neurofibromatosis is characteristically associated with self mutilation

Your answers: A.........B.........C.........D.........E.........

61. In families of schizophrenic patients

A there is an increased rate of depression

B twins are more often mentally ill than non-twins

C adoption does not reduce the genetic risk

D alcoholism occurs more often than expected

E when the proband develops the disease late in life, the risk to relatives is reduced

Your answers: A.........B.........C.........D.........E.........

62. Acute confusional states are more likely when the following conditions are present:

A hypothyroidism

B bronchopneumonia

C an unstimulating environment

D treatment with benzodiazepines

E increasing age

Your answers: A.........B.........C.........D.........E.........

Answers overleaf

60. A B

Most mental retardation is of uncertain aetiology. In mild retardation (IQ less than 50) there is a strong association with social handicap and low IQ in the family. Therefore, many cases represent the lower end of the intelligence spectrum ('subcultural' retardation). All psychiatric disorders are more common in mental retardation, although diagnosis is often difficult. Phenylketonuria requires dietary phenylalanine exclusion which can probably be ended after adolescence. Cretinism (congenital hypothyroidism) is not clinically detectable until six months. Lesch-Nyhan syndrome is an X-linked syndrome producing choreoathetoid movements and self mutilation. Neurofibromatosis is an autosomal dominant inherited disorder characterised by multiple tumours and vitiligo which only produces intellectual retardation in a minority of cases.

61. C D E

Family studies have shown that first degree relatives of schizophrenics have an increased rate of schizophrenia themselves (5-12% compared to 1% in the general population). Twin and adoption studies have confirmed the genetic contribution to aetiology. However twins per se have no greater risk than non-twins. Relatives also have higher rates of personality disorder and alcoholism but not depression or organic psychosis. Familial risk is less in late onset cases.

62. A B C D E

Most significant medical illnesses can cause confusion, particularly in the elderly where cerebral reserve may be low. It occurs more commonly in association with any form of brain damage, anxiety, understimulation and drug dependence. Myxoedema can cause many of the commonest psychiatric syndromes i.e. acute confusion, dementia, depression and paranoid psychosis.

63. Morbid jealousy (delusions of infidelity)
A is associated with hypersexuality
B is a significant cause of wife-murder
C is a recognised symptom of alcoholism
D has a good prognosis when treated early
E was attributed to unconscious homosexual urges by Freud

Your answers: A.........B.........C.........D.........E.........

64. Recognised treatments for schizophrenia include
A psychoanalysis
B chlorpromazine
C electroconvulsive treatment (ECT)
D amitriptyline
E sulpiride

Your answers: A.........B.........C.........D.........E.........

65. In combat situations
A rates of psychosis remain unchanged
B 'shell shock' is a variety of combat neurosis
C the rate of battle neurosis is higher during retreat than during attack
D fresh combat units have higher rates of psychiatric disorder
E self-inflicted wounds are more common in dangerous situations

Your answers: A.........B.........C.........D.........E.........

Answers overleaf

63. B C E

Pathological jealousy occurs in a wide range of psychiatric conditions notably personality disorder, paranoid psychosis and schizophrenia, depression and alcoholism. It is commoner in men, and is associated with erectile impotence. Freud believed it was caused by repression and reaction formation of homosexual drives. Morbid jealousy can be highly dangerous and is the cause of 10-20% of homicides in special hospitals (both male and female). Treatment of the primary disorder can be helpful but in most cases the symptom persists and marital separation may be the only solution.

64. B C D E

Schizophrenia is a complex disorder with a wide variety of presentations. In acute episodes, delusions and hallucinations respond to neuroleptic treatments like chlorpromazine, haloperidol and trifluoperazine. Sulpiride is a new antipsychotic drug which appears to cause less tardive dyskinesia. Depressive symptoms are common and may respond to antidepressive therapy e.g. amitriptyline. ECT can be valuable in intractable severe cases. Supportive psychotherapy may be helpful, but formal psychoanalysis is only indicated for neuroses and personality disorders.

65. A B D E

Combat is an extreme stressor which offers an interesting perspective on psychiatric aetiology. Psychotic disorders (such as schizophrenia) do not increase, which suggests an endogenous causation. Other psychiatric disorders increase when fighting is more severe or prolonged. Like self-inflicted wounds and desertion, they occur when most useful in avoiding danger. Moreover, only 'acceptable' symptoms are presented e.g. in World War One 'shell shock' (believed erroneously to be an organic disorder due to bomb blasts) was acceptable. In combat situations where being psychiatrically ill confers no survival advantage (e.g. patrols, retreat and naval warfare) there is no increase in neurosis. Previous combat experience and group cohesion appear to protect against neurotic breakdown.

66. **The following statements about lithium carbonate are true:**
    A it is the drug of choice in schizophrenia
    B it can be given in the form of long acting injections
    C it is known to produce increased mortality due to renal damage
    D reduction of antidiuretic hormone (ADH) levels occur in 10% of treated patients
    E it is particularly useful when rapid control of symptoms is required

    Your answers: A.........B.........C.........D.........E.........

67. **Tardive dyskinesia**
    A is associated with previous brain damage
    B occurs in most patients on long-term neuroleptic treatment
    C is commoner in men
    D is associated with reduced life expectancy in severe schizophrenia
    E invariably improves on stopping the offending neuroleptic

    Your answers: A.........B.........C.........D.........E.........

68. **The following features are characteristic of hysterical personality disorder:**
    A suggestibility
    B superficial emotional relationships
    C egocentricity
    D craving for excitement
    E globus hystericus

    Your answers: A.........B.........C.........D.........E.........

Answers overleaf

66. None are correct

Lithium carbonate is an oral medication whose main indication is to prevent relapses of bipolar manic-depressive disorder. It has a minor role as adjunctive therapy in schizophrenia and has a slow but worthwhile action on acute manic symptoms. Side-effects at therapeutic levels include; fine tremor, weight gain, thyroid enlargement and polyuria/polydipsia. The latter is due to renal unresponsiveness to normal circulating ADH levels and usually disappears on stopping treatment. Reports of chronic nephropathy are unconfirmed.

67. D

Tardive dyskinesia is characterised by chewing, sucking and grimacing of the face and choreoathetoid movements. It occurs in about one fifth of patients receiving long-term treatment with neuroleptic medication such as phenothiazines or butyrophenones. Increased incidence is seen with females and increasing age but not brain damage or previous treatment with ECT. Few treatments are helpful and stopping the offending drug may produce paradoxical worsening. There is decreased life expectancy when functional psychosis and severe dyskinesia are both present.

68. A B C D

Personality disorders are relatively stable maladaptive patterns of behaviour which cause suffering to the patient or society. Patients with hysterical personality disorder are described as egocentric, self-dramatising, attention-seeking, suggestible, manipulative and needing repeated novelty and excitement. There is a predisposition for these patients to develop conversion hysteria, which essentially consists of any of a vast range of physical symptoms caused by underlying psychological conflict or needs. Among such symptoms was thought to be 'globus hystericus' i.e. hysterical difficulty in swallowing, but recent research has shown that this symptom is almost always caused by oesophageal disease or dysfunction.

69. On general medical wards

A at least one in ten patients has depression

B medical students are better than nurses at detecting psychiatric disorder

C about one in five patients has alcohol problems

D medical outcome is affected by the presence of psychiatric disorder

E most patients who have taken a drug overdose require inpatient assessment in a psychiatric unit

Your answers: A.........B.........C.........D.........E.........

70. The following statements are true:

A psychiatric abnormalities occur more commonly in multiple sclerosis than muscular dystrophy

B in multiple sclerosis, euphoria is more frequent when disease-induced intellectual deficits are present

C the intensity of depression in Parkinson's disease correlates with the severity of movement disorder

D when depression occurs after a stroke, a lesion in the right parietal region should be strongly suspected

E the most common psychiatric presentation of neurosyphilis is dementia

Your answers: A.........B.........C.........D.........E.........

71. Monoamine oxidase inhibiting drugs (MAOIs) interact with

A Bovril

B tricyclic antidepressants

C pethidine

D phenelzine

E phentolamine

Your answers: A.........B.........C.........D.........E.........

Answers overleaf

69. A B C D

Hospital surveys have emphasised the frequency of psychiatric illness on general medical wards. The most common reason for admission is a drug overdose. Among patients admitted for other reasons, depression (10-25%) and alcohol abuse (15-30%) are very common. The diagnosis is often missed, especially if tearfulness or behaviour disturbances are not evident. This is important as continued psychiatric symptoms delay medical recovery. Research has shown that medical students can detect psychiatric cases more readily than house officers or ward nurses. About 10% of deliberate self-harm patients need inpatient psychiatric treatment.

70. A B C E

About 75% of patients with multiple sclerosis suffer from a psychiatric disorder at some stage. Euphoria and denial of disability are common associations of plaque-induced cognitive deficits, while depression is more often an early reaction to illness. Dementia and depression are also common in Parkinson's disease. There is a significant correlation between severity of depression and of the signs of Parkinson's disease. Strokes in the left frontal region are associated with depression; right parietal lesions often lead to denial of disability. Dementia and depression are both more common in neurosyphilis than the better known grandiose presentation (about 10% of cases).

71. A B C

Phenelzine is the most commonly prescribed monoamine oxidase inhibitor. Severe hypertensive crises may occur with tyramine-containing foods including cheese, meat and yeast extracts (like Bovril) and pickled herrings. Dangerous interactions may also occur with a wide range of drugs including ephedrine and phenylpropanolamine (proprietary cold remedies), methyldopa, opiates, barbiturates and tricyclic antidepressants. Some psychiatrists use combinations of MAOIs and tricyclic antidepressants to treat intractable depression, but this practice is dangerous in non-specialist hands. Phentolamine blocks alpha-adrenoceptors and is used to treat hypertensive crises induced by MAOI drugs.

72. Electroconvulsive treatment
A is known to produce long-term memory impairment in patients when compared with untreated depressives
B is not safe in patients over 80 years of age
C is of no use in neurotic depression
D is more successful in depression when delusions are present
E has been validated in double blind trials

Your answers: A.........B.........C.........D.........E.........

73. The risk of alcohol dependence is increased in
A doctors
B brewery workers
C relatives of alcoholics
D Jews
E societies with restrictive licensing laws

Your answers: A.........B.........C.........D.........E.........

74. Puerperal psychosis
A has been called 'maternity blues'
B recurs in the majority of later pregnancies
C is significantly increased after obstetric complications
D should be managed by separation of mother and baby in most cases
E may be accompanied by clouding of consciousness

Your answers: A.........B.........C.........D.........E.........

Answers overleaf

72. D E

Recent double blind trials have confirmed the particular value of electroconvulsive therapy in depression especially when endogenous features or delusions are present. Although less used in other conditions, it is of value in neurotic depression, mania and schizophrenia. It causes brief memory disturbances after each application, especially when bilateral rather than unilateral electrodes are used. However, there is little evidence that permanent memory deficits occur. Age is no contraindication to treatment.

73. A B C

Rates of alcohol consumption and dependence are higher in certain occupations including alcohol production and sales, doctors, seamen, printers, actors and sales representatives. The common characteristic appears to be availability of alcohol within relatively unsupervised routine working arrangements. Alcohol dependence is more common in countries with high average consumption; usually alcohol is cheap and licensing laws are liberal. Ethnic factors are also important with high rates in North America among negro and Irish communities and low rates in Jewish communities.

74. E

Serious and minor mental disorders are considerably more common in the postpartum period. 'Maternity blues' is a self-limiting episode of mood lability occurring in about half of new mothers. Puerperal psychosis is far less common. No specific causative factors are known. A variety of presentations are possible, including acute organic reactions with clouding of consciousness. The development of supervised mother-and-baby units within psychiatric hospitals has avoided the need for separation and the consequent disruption of emotional 'bonding'. Psychosis recurs in about 20% of later pregnancies.

75. Munchausen's syndrome is characterised by
   A female sex
   B delusions of illness
   C obsessional personality
   D folie á deux
   E recovery after surgical intervention

   Your answers: A.........B.........C.........D.........E.........

76. Delusions
   A only occur in schizophrenia
   B are not modified by contrary experience
   C are obsessions
   D are perceived as emanating from the external world
   E are false ideas

   Your answers: A.........B.........C.........D.........E.........

77. Delusions of persecution can occur in
   A paraphrenia
   B paranoid personality disorder
   C reactive depression
   D myxoedema
   E amphetamine abuse

   Your answers: A.........B.........C.........D.........E.........

Answers overleaf

75. None are correct

Patients with Munchausen's syndrome (hospital addiction) are classically males who fabricate physical and mental symptoms to obtain hospitalisation and treatment. They are evasive about their past and have psychopathic personality traits. They do not really believe themselves to be ill (unlike patients with hysteria). Prognosis is probably poor and many have repeated operations. Folie á deux refers to two people in close contact who share the same delusion. Usually one requires antipsychotic treatment while the other more submissive person recovers spontaneously when they are separated.

76. B E

Delusions are morbid false beliefs, which occur in a wide range of psychoses including schizophrenia. Classically they are firmly held out of keeping with the patient's subculture and cannot be altered by reason or demonstration of their falsity. They often occur secondary to hallucinations, which are false percepts apparently in the external world. Obsessions are recurrent thoughts, images or impulses resisted by the patient who finds them both senseless and distressing, but recognises them as his own mental products.

77. A D E

Persecutory delusions are the leading feature of paraphrenia, a psychosis typically of elderly deaf, socially isolated women with premorbid schizoid or paranoid traits. Myxoedema can produce a variety of serious mental disorders, including paranoid psychosis. Amphetamine abuse frequently produces a psychotic disorder with paranoid delusions and hallucinations, which may remit rapidly with abstinence. Patients with paranoid personalities have a pervasive sense of being slighted or tricked which does not reach delusional intensity. Persecutory delusions occur in endogenous (psychotic) depression rather than reactive depression.

78. Characteristic features of endogenous depression include
A incongruity of mood and thinking
B early morning waking
C failure to respond to chlorpromazine therapy
D feelings of worthlessness
E loss of libido

Your answers: A.........B.........C.........D.........E.........

79. Recognised features of mania include
A depression during the manic phase
B depression after recovery from the manic phase
C therapeutic response to lithium carbonate
D therapeutic response to electroconvulsive treatment (ECT)
E insomnia

Your answers: A.........B.........C.........D.........E.........

80. Recognised features of depression in the elderly include
A delusions of poverty
B pseudodementia
C a strong association with bereavement
D agitated movements
E retarded movements

Your answers: A.........B.........C.........D.........E.........

Answers overleaf

78. B D E

In endogenous depression, there is persistent depression of mood, unreactive to circumstances. Characteristic symptoms include early morning waking, morning worsening of mood, feelings of guilt or worthlessness with decline in concentration, energy, appetite, interest and libido. Although tricyclic antidepressants and electroconvulsive therapy (ECT) are the treatments of choice, some cases, especially when agitation and/or delusions are present, respond to chlorpromazine alone. Affective incongruity is a feature of schizophrenia.

79. A B C D E

Lithium carbonate is highly effective both in treating and preventing manic episodes. Occasionally in severe episodes, ECT is used. Symptoms of mania include rapid speech, hyperactivity, elevated mood, grandiose or paranoid ideas, aggression and insomnia. Most patients with mania have depressive episodes at other times in their lives. About 50% of manic patients have a sufficient admixture of depressive symptoms to qualify as depressed on standard rating scales.

80. A B D E

Agitation and retardation both occur in a significant number of elderly depressives. When delusions are present, they usually have a depressive flavour e.g. poverty or physical illness. A certain proportion have apparent cognitive deficits, which improve in parallel with the symptoms of depression: this is the commonest variety of 'pseudodementia'. Severe life events can precipitate depression in the elderly, but bereavement is less important as a cause of mental illness than in younger age groups.

81. Recognised features of anorexia nervosa include
A increased plasma cortisol
B frequent structural abnormalities of the hypothalamus
C male hypersexuality
D hypokalaemia
E total loss of body hair

Your answers: A.........B.........C.........D.........E.........

82. The following features suggest a normal bereavement reaction rather than depressive illness:
A complaints of physical symptoms
B emotional numbness
C suicidal thoughts
D searching behaviour
E feelings of worthlessness

Your answers: A.........B.........C.........D.........E.........

83. Solvent abuse
A is more common in males than females
B only causes deaths when toluene-based products are used
C may cause persistent cerebellar signs
D stops within six months in most cases
E is a cause of visual hallucinations

Your answers: A.........B.........C.........D.........E.........

Answers overleaf

81. A D

Anorexia nervosa is defined by self induced weight loss, abnormal attitudes to food and body weight and amenorrhoea in women or loss of libido in men. There are many endocrine changes e.g. raised cortisol and growth hormone, and decreased gonadotrophins. However there is little evidence that it is a primary endocrinological disorder. Structural lesions are rarely discovered. Clinical features include lanugo, a type of downy hair found on the extremities. Induced vomiting and purging to reduce weight often result in hypokalaemia.

82. A B D

Bereavement reactions are normal, but share features in common with depression such as misery, tearfulness, insomnia, poor concentration and anorexia. Other features of depression such as psychomotor retardation, delusions, suicidal thinking and generalised loss of self-esteem only rarely occur in bereavement. Physical symptoms are more commonly reported by the bereaved. Most typically, three stages of grieving can be distinguished: an initial phase of emotional numbness and unreality; secondly a mourning phase of variable length which may include experiences of the presence or voice of the deceased and searching behaviour; finally there is gradual acceptance and resolution.

83. A C D E

Solvent abuse is typically an activity of 11/16-year-old boys who experiment in groups. Three quarters stop abusing solvents within six months. A small number of severe chronic abusers may suffer a variety of ill effects. Glue sniffers can be detected by the smell of their breath, glue on hands and clothes and a characteristic facial rash. Acute effects include subjective euphoria, dizziness, slurred speech, impaired judgement and sometimes visual hallucinations. Chronic effects include a persistent cerebellar syndrome, cerebral ventricular enlargement and peripheral neuropathy (due to n-hexane only). Deaths are usually from cardiac arrhythmias caused by freons (aerosol propellants) rather than toluene.

84. **The following symptoms are often held to be of 'first rank' importance in making the diagnosis of schizophrenia:**
    A paranoid delusions
    B thoughts inserted into the patient's mind
    C voices in the third person commenting on the patient's actions
    D visual hallucinations
    E ideas of reference

    Your answers: A.........B.........C.........D.........E.........

85. **The following statements about hyperkinetic children are correct:**
    A the diagnosis is made more often in the United States than in Britain
    B impaired attention is characteristic
    C the condition usually abates at puberty
    D benzodiazepines are often helpful
    E treatment with amphetamines runs the considerable risk of later drug abuse

    Your answers: A.........B.........C.........D.........E.........

86. **The following factors are associated with physical abuse of a child (non-accidental injury):**
    A age under two years
    B obstetric complications
    C poor mothering ability noted in the postnatal ward
    D criminality in the parents
    E illegitimacy

    Your answers: A.........B.........C.........D.........E.........

Answers overleaf

84. B C

'First rank' symptoms are often used by psychiatrists to diagnose schizophrenia. They include passivity experiences (i.e. thoughts, feelings or actions experienced as 'made' by external agencies); thought insertion, withdrawal or broadcasting; delusional perception, a complex form of primary delusion; and three particular types of auditory hallucination, in the third person, running commentary and having one's thoughts spoken aloud. Paranoid delusions, visual hallucinations and ideas of reference all occur in schizophrenia but are not of particular diagnostic significance.

85. A B C

Problems of definition mean that American psychiatrists diagnose up to 4% of children as hyperkinetic, while their British counterparts use a much narrower concept, i.e. pervasive restlessness, motor overactivity, poor attention and impulsiveness. The condition usually disappears at puberty except when it is very severe and/or intellectual retardation is also present. Benzodiazepines and barbiturates are contraindicated as they produce paradoxical disinhibition. Amphetamines can cause growth retardation and appetite suppression but not subsequent drug abuse.

86. A B C D E

Physical harm or serious neglect of children tends to occur in parents with one or more of these characteristics: personality disorder, low social class, criminality, mental illness, marital disharmony and abuse in their own childhood. Abused children are generally under two years old. Certain features increase the risk of abuse: complications in pregnancy or labour, separation from mother in postnatal period, congenital defects and persistent crying. Even bearing in mind these factors, prediction of later child abuse is difficult: hospital observation of mothering skills after delivery may be a useful indicator.

87. When persistent absences are due to school refusal

A entry into secondary school may trigger onset of the problem

B most cases require a behavioural programme

C there is an association with specific reading retardation

D the majority develop adult neurosis

E there is more neurosis in the family than would be expected by chance

Your answers: A.........B.........C.........D.........E.........

88. Recognised features of chronic schizophrenia include

A pressure of speech

B age disorientation

C self-dramatisation

D good response to chlorpromazine

E ventricular enlargement shown by air encephalography

Your answers: A.........B.........C.........D.........E.........

89. Prolonged benzodiazepine use

A occurs in almost 1% of British adults

B is no more effective than brief counselling in minor neurotic disorders

C produces rapid tolerance to hypnotic effects

D can lead to a withdrawal syndrome

E is associated with shoplifting

Your answers: A.........B.........C.........D.........E.........

Answers overleaf

87. A E

School refusal starts at three stages: between 5 and 7 years, at 11 years and over 14 years. Compared with truants, school refusers are more depressed, passive and academically successful. Specific reading retardation is often associated with truancy and other conduct disorders. Most cases, especially in younger age groups, respond to a sympathetically arranged return to school. Only the most severe cases need psychological treatment programmes and of these, only about one-third develop neurotic symptoms in adult life.

88. B E

The most typical symptoms of chronic schizophrenia are social withdrawal, reduced activity and speech, and odd or self-neglectful behaviour. Recent research has revealed a subgroup of chronic institutionalised schizophrenics with cerebral ventricular enlargement and minor cognitive deficits, notably a tendency to markedly underestimate age and length of hospitalisation. Self-dramatisation is a common feature of hysterical personality disorder. Marked pressure of speech may indicate the presence of mania.

89. B C D E

It has been estimated that 3 million people in the United Kingdom are chronic users of benzodiazepines and perhaps half a million of these are dependent. Rapid tolerance develops for hypnotic and anti-convulsant effects and rather more slowly for anxiolytic effects. Periods of treatment should be short and for minor neurotic disorders, brief counselling has been shown to be equally effective. Chronic use can cause sedation, apathy, depression and disinhibition leading to paradoxical anger or uncharacteristic acts including shoplifting. The withdrawal syndrome may be severe and last for months and, in most cases, does not represent a recurrence of the original anxiety symptoms.

90. Neuroleptic malignant syndrome

    A is characterised by hyperthermia and muscular rigidity

    B can occur when tricyclics alone are administered

    C most commonly occurs after haloperidol treatment

    D is usually fatal

    E responds to treatment with tetrabenzine

    Your answers: A.........B.........C.........D.........E.........

91. In patients who have taken an overdose of tablets, later completed suicide is made more likely by the presence of

    A male sex

    B precautions to avoid discovery

    C early parental loss

    D past history of endogenous depression

    E a diagnosis of schizophrenia

    Your answers: A.........B.........C.........D.........E.........

92. The following factors are significantly associated with episodes of deliberate self harm:

    A male unemployment

    B recent alcohol consumption

    C male sex

    D age over 40 years

    E epilepsy

    Your answers: A.........B.........C.........D.........E.........

Answers overleaf

90. A B C

Neuroleptic malignant syndrome is an uncommon but increasingly recognised side effect of neuroleptic administration. The syndrome is characterised by hyperthermia, muscle rigidity, a fluctuant conscious level, features of sympathetic discharge and, less consistently, dystonias and dyskinesias. It occurs at therapeutic doses. The most frequently implicated drug is haloperidol. Tricyclic antidepressant therapy and L-dopa withdrawal are occasional causes. There is no specific treatment. A significant minority of cases are fatal; the rest recover after drug withdrawal within one to three weeks.

91. A B D E

Studies of parasuicide have shown that eventual suicide is predicted by evidence of serious intent (precautions against discovery, planning, dangerous method, writing a suicide note or making a will); previous suicide attempts; the presence of depressive illness, alcoholism, drug abuse or antisocial personality disorder; male sex, older age, unemployment and social isolation. Lifetime risk of suicide is 15% in endogenous depression and probably about 10% in schizophrenia.

92. A B E

The most typical pattern of deliberate self harm is an impulsive drug overdose taken with mixed motives in a state of mental turmoil often by a young single girl after a quarrel or rejection. Important associations include recent life events, marital conflict, unemployment (in men), recent alcohol consumption (especially in men), personality disorder and epilepsy. In the year following an overdose, risk of suicide is 1-2% (100 times that of the general population).

93. Recognised features of Korsakov's syndrome include
A denial of amnesia
B impaired registration rather than retention
C obsession with time
D dysphasia
E echopraxia

Your answers: A.........B.........C.........D.........E.........

94. In encopresis (faecal soiling)
A boys are more often affected than girls
B children with 'aggressive' soiling are often clean in other aspects of their life
C 'regressive' soiling has a better prognosis than 'aggressive' soiling
D Hirschsprung's disease should be excluded
E tricyclic antidepressants can be helpful

Your answers: A.........B.........C.........D.........E.........

95. Nocturnal enuresis
A occurs in 1% of teenagers
B is associated with psychiatric disorder in the majority of cases
C is associated with abnormally deep sleep
D occurs in non-REM sleep
E runs in families

Your answers: A.........B.........C.........D.........E.........

Answers overleaf

93. A

Korsakov's syndrome is characterised by relatively circumscribed memory deficit where new information is registered but quickly forgotten. This results in disorientation in time. Patients usually have little awareness of their problem and make up stories (confabulate) to cover gaps in their memory. Associations include irritability, peripheral neuropathy and the Wernicke syndrome (ataxia, ophthalmoplegia and impaired consciousness). Common aetiologies are thiamine deficiency (due to alcohol abuse or gastrointestinal disease) and lesions of the mammillary bodies and medial thalamus. Echopraxia (automatic imitation of another's movements) is a symptom of catatonia.

94. A B C D

Faecal soiling is called encopresis when physical cases such as faecal impaction with overflow and Hirschsprung's disease have been excluded. About 80% of cases occur in boys. 'Aggressive' and 'regressive' types of emotional disorder have been described. In the former case, a typical presentation would be revolt against a controlling parent with scrupulous cleanliness in other activities. In 'regressive' soiling, there has often been a traumatic life event and rapid improvement is the general rule. Tricyclic antidepressants are useful in nocturnal enuresis but in encopresis would merely cause constipation.

95. A D E

Nocturnal enuresis decreases steadily with increasing age, affecting about 10% at age 5 and 1% at age 15. 70% of affected children have a first degree relative who has also been affected. Psychiatric disorder is not found in most cases, but if present suggests a worse prognosis. Voiding occurs in non-REM sleep, but no abnormal sleep pattern has been found.

96. The following features are more likely to occur in depressive pseudodementia than in dementia:

A recent onset of symptoms
B extensive complaining by the patient about memory loss
C worsening of cognitive symptoms in the evening
D 'don't know' answers
E past history of depression

Your answers: A.........B.........C.........D.........E.........

97. In tuberose sclerosis (epiloia)

A autosomal dominant inheritance is usual
B epilepsy often occurs
C a significant minority of cases has normal intelligence
D cherry red spot at the macula of the retina is a useful distinguishing feature
E male patients frequently have enlarged testes

Your answers: A.........B.........C.........D.........E.........

98. Fetal alcohol syndrome

A is a recognised cause of hyperkinetic behaviour
B occurs in most pregnancies where the mother drinks over 400 ml of wine per day
C is a common cause of severe mental retardation
D includes microcephaly and epicanthic folds
E may not be completely attributable to alcohol

Your answers: A.........B.........C.........D.........E.........

Answers overleaf

96. **A B D E**

The differential diagnosis of dementia and depression can be troublesome when cognitive symptoms complicate the latter. In depression, careful questioning will typically elicit more recent onset and more rapid progression of symptoms and possibly a past history or family history of depression. Features of the mental state suggesting depression include complaints about memory loss, 'don't know' rather than 'near miss' answers to specific questions and concurrent depressive symptoms. All these features are less common in dementia. In depression there is morning worsening of mood while in dementia there is evening worsening of confusion.

97. **A B C**

Tuberose sclerosis is caused by an autosomal dominant gene of variable penetrance. Mental retardation occurs in two thirds of cases and therefore normal intelligence is found in a significant minority of cases. Features include epilepsy, adenoma sebaceum, white skin patches and shagreen skin, intracerebral calcification and cataracts. Cherry red macular spots occur in Tay-Sachs disease, while enlarged testes are strongly associated with X-linked mental retardation.

98. **A D E**

The fetal alcohol syndrome includes facial abnormalities (including microcephaly, prominent forehead, maxillary hypoplasia, and epicanthic folds), low birth weight, mental retardation, failure to thrive and hyperkinetic behaviour. It occurs in 1-2 per 1000 births and characteristically mental retardation is mild or moderate. Prospective research has shown that when pregnant mothers drink excessively, low birth weight and stillbirths are more common than the full syndrome. Mothers who drink heavily also often have other risk factors (e.g. smoking, malnutrition and social handicaps) which may have aetiological significance.

99. Huntington's chorea

A is caused by an X-linked gene

B is the commonest cause of choreiform movements first occurring in the second half of life

C is associated with decreased glutamic acid decarboxylase (GAD)

D particularly affects the cerebral cortex and basal ganglia

E causes rapidly progressive dementia in the majority of cases

Your answers: A.........B.........C.........D.........E.........

100. The following features are found in the majority of cases of Down's syndrome:

A IQ between 20 and 50

B death before the age of 50 years

C congenital heart disease

D behaviour disorder

E flat occiput

Your answers: A.........B.........C.........D.........E.........

Answers overleaf

99. C D

Huntington's chorea is an uncommon autosomal dominant disorder affecting 4-7 per 100,000 of the population. Senile and drug induced choreas are much more frequently encountered. Anatomically, the frontal lobes and the caudate nucleus are most severely affected by neuronal loss and gliosis. Decreased concentrations of the inhibitory transmitter gamma-amino-butyric acid (GABA) and its enzyme glutamic acid decarboxylase (GAD) are usually detected. Dementia is usual although not invariable and progresses slowly over five to fifteen years.

100. A B E

Down's syndrome is the commonest known cause of moderate or severe subnormality (IQ less than 50). Characteristic features include small mouth with furrowed tongue and high palate, flat occiput, eyes with oblique palpebral fissures and epicanthic folds, hypotonia, short broad hands with curved little finger and a single palmar crease. Congenital heart disease (especially septal defects) occur in one fifth of cases. Behaviour disorders are less common than in many syndromes of mental handicap. Despite improvements in care, death in early or middle life is still usual.

REVISION INDEX

Each item in this index refers to a specific question or answer. The numbers given refer to question numbers not page numbers.